Motherhood Is a B#tch!

Praise for Lyss Stern and *Motherhood is a B#tch!*

"Her hilarious writing will make you laugh out loud, but, more importantly, it will make you feel understood. Don't listen to the mommy noise. Follow your gut, do the best you can, and 'lyssen' to Lyss!"

—Jill Kargman, author and creator and star of Odd Mom Out

"Finally, a book that doesn't sugarcoat the idea of what it is to be a mother. Basically, we are f#cking warriors."

—Rebecca Minkoff, fashion designer

"Lyss tells it like it is while making us laugh at all the craziness and chaos that is motherhood. Her message is empowering—go forth and be fierce! Her book is an eye-opener that every modern mom needs to read!"

—Kelly Rutherford, actress

"Lyss represents every mom in her quest to do it all in a 'fabulyss' way! She's savvy, strong, smart, sexy, and confident. But her most appealing trait is her passion for helping other moms find the tools within themselves to create their own 'fabulyss' worlds."

—Jenny Hutt, host of Just Jenny on Sirius XM Satellite Radio

"There's much to be admired about Lyss Stern. [She's] tireless with a strength and purpose to help other women who secretly struggle. She's a beautiful person who puts her vanity aside to just make us all feel empowered . . . and that's something to be applauded."

—Sasha Charnin Morrison, pop culture connoisseur and author of Secrets of Stylists

"Nobody tells you that [the] giggling baby in the Ivory Snow commercial is never going to let you sleep. Nobody tells you [that the] adorable toddler in bows is going to come home one day with a nose ring ... Lyss tells you what nobody else will while showing you how to be the most 'fabulyss' mom, wife, and success you can be!

—Erika Katz, author of Bonding Over Beauty

"Wait, I know your husband. Is that him on the front cover?? (I'm never letting him forget this.)"

—Samantha Bee, comedian, writer, producer, political commentator, and host of Full Frontal

"We all lose ourselves when we enter the sisterhood of motherhood. So, let's laugh, learn, and embrace the moments together. After all, there is perfection in the imperfection."

—Sukanya Krishnan, lead anchor of PIX11 Morning News and five-time Emmy Award winner

Motherhood Is a B#tch!

10 Steps to Regaining Your Sanity, Sexiness, and Inner Diva

by Lyss Stern
with Sheryl Berk

Foreword by Jill Kargman

Skyhorse Publishing books may be purchased in bulk at special discounts for sales promotion, corporate gifts, fund-raising, or educational purposes. Special editions can also be created to specifications. For details, contact the Special Sales Department, Skyhorse Publishing, 307 West 36th Street, 11th Floor, New York, NY 10018 or info@skyhorsepublishing.com.

Skyhorse® and Skyhorse Publishing® are registered trademarks of Skyhorse Publishing, Inc.®, a Delaware corporation.

Visit our website at www.skyhorsepublishing.com.

10 9 8 7 6 5 4 3 2 1

Library of Congress Cataloging-in-Publication Data is available on file.

Cover design by Bonnie Marcus Collection

Print ISBN: 978-1-5107-1897-5
Ebook ISBN: 978-1-5107-1896-8

Printed in the United States of America

This book is designed to provide information and motivation to readers. It is sold with the understanding that the authors are not engaged to render any type of psychological, health, fitness, or any other kind of professional advice. Consult your doctor or physician before starting any type of fitness routine.

This book is dedicated to my three children:
Jackson, Oliver, and BlakeyBleu.
You have given me the strength to write this book for all
the moms out there in the world
who need to find their voice and breathe!
And to my loving husband, Brian,
who always says "yes," even when he should be saying "no."

CONTENTS

FOREWORD

I was a loner mom. When I shat out my now-teenager, I had no friends with babies. I pushed the stroller solo, observing the preened cliques of bedecked mothers and their perfect offspring. The girls' grosgrain bows were large enough to be helicopter propellers. The boys were not sandbox filthy and wore lederhosen. The moms had designer diaper bags containing little Ziploc bags of cut-up grapes, diapers lined up like soldiers, and an extra-squeaky giraffe.

I always felt sloppy or weird in my black ensembles that looked like Urban Outfitters threw up on me, while the Lilly Pulitzer army was pulled together flawlessly. They had every hair in place and my nonkeratin'd jewfro was frizzing to Staten Island. Their kids were counting to ten—in French—and my daughter would yell something about vaginas.

I endured raised eyebrows and dirty looks when I gave my kids something that fell on the floor (five-second rule!), and I often felt like everyone else's homes were immaculate and perfect, while mine looked like it was walloped by a Fisher-Price cyclone.

But then one day I turned a corner. I realized that if the grass is always greener, it's probably AstroTurf. It's a mirage, a barely cobbled-together snapshot that unravels when they go home. Or, they have half of Manila in their penthouse, bolstering them. Or, they actually ARE perfect . . . but the kids are so micromanaged and controlled they may be fuckups later. Who knows. What I do know and appreciate is candor. When I met Lyss Stern, our kids were in kindergarten. I knew I was in the presence of a real mother and not a fembot construct. We didn't use baby talk or never lose our cool. We didn't have hot and cold running help. We commiserated about our kids' silly behavior in music class, our exhaustion, our desire to bring back the fabulosity, or should I say "fabu*lyss*ity"!?

With Divamoms, she created a touchstone for busy city mothers to connect and peel back the bullshit. To get a break, a drink, a moment out of the house during what most people call Happy Hour, but mothers know it is actually Crappy Hour.

Years before I had my TV show, *Odd Mom Out*, she celebrated me and my books, and I will never forget it. She celebrates other women and understands the communal aspect of honesty and speaking up, swapping horror stories, and, above all, laughing.

Her hilarious writing will make you laugh out loud, but, more importantly, it will make you feel understood. The only problem with this book is that I wish I'd had it fourteen years ago—it's a comforting chorus of the voice I only experienced in my head. I would've felt a little less stressed about all the mommy noise of "you have to get into this class," or "everyone is going to this pediatrician to the stars," or "you must do this or your kid will wind up in jail." Don't listen to any of it. Follow your gut, do the best you can, and *lyssen* to Lyss.

—*Jill Kargman*

INTRODUCTION

Once upon a time there was a girl who loved her career, her body, her friends, her life. She went to yoga and spin class five times a week; she never missed an episode of *Scandal* or an issue of *Vogue*. She looked fabulous and felt invincible.

Fast-forward twenty years: that "princess" is now frumpy, frazzled, and baking banana bread at 5:00 a.m. for her son's fourth-grade class. She can't remember the last time she got her hair colored, her nails done, or had time to pee. (Was it yesterday?) She looks in the mirror and doesn't recognize the person staring back at her. What happened? Where did she go? Was she abducted by aliens? The Demogorgon on *Stranger Things*?

Sound familiar? Welcome to my world. For the longest time, I thought I was living a freakin' fairy tale in reverse. I felt out of control, out of sorts, and out of my mind. How did other moms manage to be so put-together? What did they have that I didn't have? "Kelly Ripa ... Beyoncé ... JLo," I pleaded to the TV screen, "what is your secret, you BITCH?"

I would cry and complain to anyone who would listen, which is exactly how this book came about. One morning, when I went to grab coffee with a friend, I had an epiphany. As we stood there, waiting for the barista to whip up something extra-large and extra-strong to pry my eyes open at 8:00 a.m., I launched into my usual tirade, bemoaning my lack of sleep, lack of sex, lack of a life *period*. "Motherhood is a b#tch!" I proclaimed, maybe a little too loudly. Then it dawned on me, if that were the case, then that's what I needed to become: a bitch—and not just a little one, mind you. I had to become a woman who kicked ass and took no prisoners. I needed to fight back against anyone who has ever sugarcoated what mothers go through on a daily basis (just about every motherhood book out there). I was sick and tired and not gonna take it anymore.

All the way home, I pondered the question: could I find a way back to the woman that I once was and still be a great mother, wife, and class parent? Could I get my act together and stop smelling like *eau de spit-up*? Could I ban elastic waistbands from my wardrobe and make my husband and kids treat me as more than just chief cook and bottle washer? Could I stop the endless cycle of exhaustion and exasperation? As Sarah Palin (bitchy mama extraordinaire) would say, "You betcha!"

So, here's the bad news: there's no fairy godmother out there for harried moms on the verge of a nervous breakdown. If there were, someone would have hired her years ago and given her a reality TV show. Now for the good news: you don't need a magic wand to transform yourself from a pumpkin into a human being. Just follow the ten easy steps in this book in order to up your game and regain your life.

Get off your ass and start bitchin'!

Being a bitch is not about ranting, raving, or ripping someone's head off for the fun of it (but, hey, don't knock it till you've tried it). It's about confidence and control and knowing when and where to dig your four-inch heels into the ground. It's about standing up for yourself and giving voice to your needs and feelings. It's about asking for help and demanding support when you're at the end of your rope (which, in my case, is daily). And, you don't need Beyoncé's bank account to do it. Truly, it's not about the money, honey. It's about the 'tude.

People may call you a bitch. So what. If they don't say it, they're probably thinking it. Why? Because women are supposed to be sacrificing all the time. They're supposed to mama martyrs. If you're not, then clearly you *must* be a bitch. And therein lies the problem: most people say "bitch" like it's a bad thing. Why? Because they don't want you to make changes and stir things up. They don't want you to assert yourself—that's threatening to them. The world isn't supportive of bitchy moms.

And, sometimes, the very people we thought would always back us up (spouses, friends, relatives) let us down the most. Disappointment is a bitch, too.

But once you become a full-fledged bitch, everything changes. People see you differently. When they're looking for a patsy or a pushover, they have to set their sights elsewhere. When they want to be critical or catty, they must think twice before opening their mouths. When they see you coming, they step aside and pay you the R-E-S-P-E-C-T you deserve. Yes, Aretha, there is a Santa Claus. I'm giving you this amazing, powerful, earthshaking gift. You are gonna be one happy, healthy bitch with family, friends, and frenemies alike falling at your feet. You're going to look good, feel good, walk proud, and never, ever apologize. Trust me, I was in your playground-friendly shoes (you know, the Aerosoles loafers with the memory foam insole) not that long ago. I know it's hard. I know it takes cojones. But you can, and you will, do it. There are no more options. This is reality calling, and it's time for you to answer; you simply can't live like this anymore. It's them or you.

Stop saying, "I can't, because . . ." and start saying, "How can I make this happen?" Seek out the choices that put you on the path to where you want to be. I mean that sincerely: the power is in your hands and no one else's. Marianne Williamson wrote, "Our deepest fear is not that we are inadequate. Our deepest fear is that we are powerful beyond measure." So, I dare you: be powerful beyond measure. Be bold! Go forth and be a bitch!

Quiz: Do you have bitchy mama potential?

1. A mom grabs you in the schoolyard and asks if you "wouldn't mind" watching her kid . . . for the next three hours. Her nanny phoned in sick, and she has a shrink appointment and some errands to run. The correct response is:

   a) Of course, I'll watch him! We mentally ill people have to stick together!

b) Sure, I don't mind at all. Would Billy like to stay for dinner?

c) I'm sorry. All playdates need to be arranged at least twenty-four hours in advance. Clearly you mistake me for someone without a life.

2. Your husband gets the AmEx bill and flips out over how much you spent this month. You reply:

a) Perhaps Babies"R"Us will give me diapers, wipes, and formula for free if I ask, "pretty please."

b) You're right, honey. I'll start coupon clipping tomorrow.

c) No prob . . . I'll just return that sexy new lingerie I bought to wear for you this weekend.

3. Your mother-in-law remarks that you look like you've gained some weight. You answer:

a) Gee, Mom, I guess giving birth to twins will do that to ya.

b) You're right. I should hit the gym more often.

c) Have you looked in a mirror lately?

4. The PTA in your kid's school needs someone to organize a bake sale. You say:

a) As long as you're not worried about that little food poisoning incident the last time.

b) I'm so flattered!

c) I'd love to, but I have a root canal scheduled for that day. And, frankly, it's more appealing.

5. Your babysitter asks for a raise after six months. You reply:

a) My baby sleeps for six of the eight hours you work for me. I'm sure you're severely underpaid.

b) How much do you want? I'll get my wallet; please don't leave me!

c) There are a dozen "nanny position wanted" flyers on the supermarket bulletin board. You sure you wanna be going down this road?

Answer key:

Mostly As—You're a woman who keeps her bitchiness bottled up. You have potential, but you need to let it fly! You tend to hide behind snarky remarks rather than saying what you want/feel. Your anger is bubbling under the surface, and that's just not healthy. One day you're going to explode. Say what you mean, mean what you say, and begin the 10-step program today!

Mostly Bs—You must like shoes, because clearly you are a doormat. How much abuse can one woman take? Are you trying to be fifty shades of pathetic? Honey, stop suffering and start standing up for yourself! You need to begin with step one and learn how to make your life a whole lot easier. I feel your pain, truly I do. Time to bitch.

Mostly Cs—Now you're talkin', girlfriend. You've got a mighty mouth and lots of natural bitchiness in you. Brava! Now you just need to hone those skills so people aren't offended, but they're putty in your hands. Read on.

STEP 1
EMBRACE THE BITCH

"We need to reshape our own perception of how we view ourselves. We have to step up as women and take the lead."

—*Beyoncé*

You *bitch*. Some women are so afraid of the word, they can't even say it. Besides its original meaning (a female dog), it commonly refers to a woman who is overly aggressive, rude, and belligerent. Some women get offended when they're called a bitch. I say bring it on! Being a bitch is every smart woman's birthright. I'm not interested in being Miss Congeniality anymore. I want to be Miss Bitchy Mama, crown and all. She's a woman who feels sexier, stronger, and more gorgeous *after* she has a baby. A woman who understands that loving your child doesn't mean hating yourself, and that being a mother can be the most fabulous time of your life. It's not about stepping on other people or cursing like a New York City cab driver (though, don't knock it 'til you've tried it). It's about working hard for what you want and not settling for less. It's about being self-determined instead of always self-sacrificing. A bitch is not less feminine. *Au contraire!* She has sex appeal and femininity up the wazoo! She just knows how to play those cards to her advantage.

You have a bitch in you, I promise. And maybe you've finally been pushed to the breaking point and are ready to learn how to set her free. Brava! They don't teach you this in college. I also don't want you to think this book will turn you into some heartless, evil wench. Bitches are not evil. They're smart. They're in control. They're not mean (just maybe a little snarky). I want you to redefine the word "bitch" and own it!

Let me spell it out for you.

Be the woman you want. Visualize her. The first step to your bitchy mama metamorphosis is channeling the vibe. Get your head in the game, girlfriend. If you think "I am a doormat," you will be a doormat. If you believe, "I am queen of the world," you will rock a regal attitude in everything you do.

Initiate. Saying you're going to change is nice, but useless (kind of like that Snuggie you got for Christmas). You need to actually take some action. Baby steps, babe. One day at a time. Lay out a list of how you are going to do things differently. For me, it started with getting my ass back to the gym at least once a week. That was doable. Making just one small move in the right direction will get you on the right track.

Time-out. This is one of the most important rules of being a bitch: give yourself a time-out whenever you need it. You'll learn later how (and how often) you should indulge and pamper your body and soul, but for starters, take 10 minutes out of every day to simply **breathe**. Mommies don't have a time-out chair where they can go to de-stress and quiet their minds. I've been known to hide in my walk-in closet. When you need some downtime, take it. Don't apologize. Don't feel guilty. Park your kids in front of the TV and go in your room and stare at the ceiling for a few minutes.

Care. Mommies are nurturers; we care about and for everyone in our lives. But what about ourselves? I want you to *care* that your nail polish is chipped, *care* that your scale says you gained five pounds in a week, *care* that you haven't seen a movie (*Finding Dory* doesn't count) in months. Do not sweep your needs under the rug because you're so busying taking care of everyone else. Make yourself a priority, too.

Help. Ask for it. Demand it. Hire it. You are not freakin' Superwoman, able to leap monkey bars in a single bound while changing a diaper. For God's sake, get yourself an extra pair of hands. If you can't afford a sitter or a nanny, then ask your relatives and/or neighbors to pitch in. Divvy up duties with Dad—oh yes, he can do a load of laundry, too. Get over the whole I-can-do-it-all-by-myself crap. You can't. You shouldn't. You don't have to. Bitchy moms know when to send out an SOS. Martyrdom is not flattering on anyone.

Time for a new mind-set

Think of it as a little bitchy brainwashing. First off, I want you to look in the mirror—ignore the roots and wrinkles and Cheerios stuck to your shirt—and see the potential. Don't avoid your reflection; she's not just your friend, she's your cheerleader.

Now, repeat after me, "I'm a bitch and I'm proud of it!" I like to think of it as flipping the bitch switch. Madonna had the right idea when she said, "I'm tough. I'm ambitious. I know exactly what I want. If that makes me a bitch, okay." Oh, it's more than okay, Madge. It's necessary.

You don't have to feel disheveled and downtrodden on a daily basis. You don't have to be a self-sacrificing doormat who puts everyone and everything before her own personal needs. You don't have to walk around feeling whipped and saying, "woe is me." This is your moment to take back your life—push and shove those oppressors out of the way and grab it if you have to! Acknowledge that you are a wonderful woman: brilliant, beautiful, badass. When you can look in the mirror and see that in your reflection (or at the very least, the potential), then you're ready to take the steps.

I spent a few years in therapy. There, I said it. Although not a lot of women will talk about it (as if paying to bitch is a bad thing), so have they. Go ahead, take a survey: How many women do you know who are popping antidepressants and/or Ativan like candy? How many of them have a shrink on speed dial? More than you think. Why? Because we're unhappy. We're stressed to the breaking point. We may smile, but it's all bull. I'm grinning from ear to ear right now, and I'm pissed as hell that my kid is interrupting me while I'm trying to write for five freakin' minutes! But I'm smiling!

We've become really good at faking it (and I don't mean in the sack, but yeah, that, too). We don't want anyone to know how fed up and miserable we are. If you say your life sucks, doesn't that mean you're a failure? No, it means you're human. You know it shouldn't be like this. But maybe you're stuck: you don't know how to break the cycle. You think that if you do, the foundation will crack and you'll let everyone down. Not so; they'll all survive just dandy. Don't guilt yourself into thinking this is what your life has to be.

So, what *did* I learn from my therapy sessions? That I need to be heard. Instead of bottling up my feelings, I need to talk about them and have someone actually *hear me*. Once those feelings were uttered (several times, very loudly), I felt a whole lot better. I felt relevant. I felt acknowledged. Too bad I had to pay someone $200 an hour to listen!

Now it's your turn to give a voice to your feelings. Say it loud and proud. Say that you're sick of the life you're living and the garbage that is dumped on you. No more. No. More. It's like going to an AA meeting: "Hi, my name is Lyss, and I'm a bitch." Own it. People may stop and stare; they may inch away. Good, let 'em. They won't screw with you anymore. They won't dump their kids or their thankless tasks on you. They won't ask you to get dinner on the table when you're ready to drop from exhaustion. They won't nag or needle or nudge you to death. They'll tread carefully because you mean business. You scare them. You're a force to be reckoned with. No one pushes you around because you push back. You're going to build yourself up so no one can ever tear you down again. Ever.

Believe me, I wasn't always this cool and confident. Maybe I started out that way, when I was young and in my twenties and convinced that I could have it all. I could be a mom, a wife, a working woman with a hot career! But that was three kids and twenty years ago. Now I know better. I can't be a consummate professional with a three-year-old wrapped around one leg and a dog peeing on the other one. I can't bake cupcakes for my son's class, eat one, and not have it show up on my ass later than night. I was lying to myself in thinking that I could stay the person I was. My metabolism slowed down, my boobs fell down, and my skinny jeans became a laughable misnomer. Besides the physical, there's the mental: motherhood is crazy. Batshit crazy. The chaos you go through every day would make grown men weep. Why do you think our husbands let us handle it—they don't have the balls (well, technically they do, but you know what I mean).

Shortly after my daughter's second birthday, I was feeling lousy. My body was literally trying to tell me, "Wake up! You can't live like this anymore." I went on a health retreat. That's right, out of sheer desperation (and terrified of invasive tests and procedures that my doctor seemed to think I was headed for), I packed my bags and left my husband in charge. I figured, what's the worst he can do? Set the apartment on fire? Lose my toddler in the park? Let him freakin' figure it out. For a few glorious days, I sipped tea and took herbs, ate quinoa and kiwi, and did sunrise yoga. Guess what. I came home feeling like a new person. Why? Because I paid attention to myself. I stopped putting everyone else's needs, wants, and whines before my own basic necessities: peace, love, and more than two hours of sleep. I felt renewed and rejuvenated, and my health bounced back.

My doctor was shocked. He asked, "What did you do?" I became a bitch, that's what I did. I realized this was what had to happen all the time, not just for a weekend. My husband and children kissed and hugged me when I walked through the door—they appreciated me more because they realized that without me, their lives were a mess and there was no clean underwear. Damn straight! I deserve to be appreciated, heck, worshiped. Within minutes, they tried to suck me back in: "Mommy, we need this. Honey, I need that." Well, you know what I need? I need all of you—and all the rest of you who have been driving me down this dangerous spiral of stress and self-loathing—to back the hell off. Yes, I will be a loving mother and wife, a devoted daughter, sister, and school community member, but on my terms. I'm not the same girl I was, that's for sure. But for the first time in a long time, I'm okay. Better. Stronger. I knew that going forward, I would assert myself instead of shutting my mouth for fear of disappointing someone. I was always so concerned about hurting people's feelings. Excuse me, what about *my* feelings? Don't I count? You bet I do.

And so do you. You're nodding your head—yeah, you've been there, done this. You know what I'm talking about. You know you've wanted to run away from home, not once, not twice, but every time your teenage son slams the door in your face (and that's several times a day). You feel like your husband doesn't hear you, see you, respect you as an equal. The only reason he calls you during the day is to ask what's for dinner (here's a clue: takeout!). Your boss doesn't care what you've got going on at home—that's your problem. Your mother-in-law tells you that you're doing everything wrong—or at least not as well as she would do it. And your fellow moms spot you in the schoolyard and think, "Sucker! Playdate at her house!"

Stand tall. Throw your shoulders back, boobs out. Give them the death stare. It's a start—you're a bitch in training. The words will come later. For now, silence is golden. It speaks volumes. It intimidates. All bitches are experts at the "glare like you don't care." Do not, I repeat, do not get into an argument, try to explain, defend, or excuse yourself. Bitches don't beg. They don't backpedal, and they don't *ever* let someone get the better of them. Cool as a cucumber—get it printed on a T-shirt and wear it every day if you need reminding. Lose your temper or your shit, and, I promise you, they've already won. Be the bitch you want to be. Embody her in your demeanor, your posture, your voice. Try it, it's scary stuff. When someone is putting you down or pushing your buttons, look them straight in the eye and don't blink. Don't breathe. (Think Hillary Clinton or Hannibal Lecter.) They'll either realize you're not a pushover or think you're a serial killer—either one in fine. This little maneuver works on everyone, from pushy

PTA presidents to midtantrum toddlers. When I give my dog Jedi the bitch look, he literally rolls over and plays dead. It's *that* good.

I want you to understand that this is a process. It doesn't happen overnight. It begins with thinking and believing, and then it manifests itself in how you act and react. Eventually, you'll eat, sleep, and breathe bitch. It becomes second nature. And what makes me the person to lead you on this journey? I'm one of you. I fight every day to keep it together, to be happy and healthy, mentally, physically, and emotionally. It's not a privilege; it's our right. I don't know how I wound up where I wound up, but it literally scared the living daylights out of me. I looked lousy, I felt lousy, and when I woke up in the morning, my head kept repeating, "Dread, dread, dread" when I ticked off everything I had to get done. Then I did it; I flipped the switch. I changed my way of thinking and living, and the rest fell into place. People saw me differently. They treated me differently. And I saw myself differently. I knew this was the beginning of a whole new me— and now, it's the beginning of a whole new you.

It would be selfish of me not to share; we bitches have to stick together.

---

5 Bitchy Mantras to Recite Every Day

Look in that mirror and say it like you mean it:

"I am bitch, hear me roar."

"Bitches rule the world."

"Did you just call me a bitch? So glad you noticed."

"Karma won't be a bitch if you are."

"Life's a bitch—but I'm bitchier."

Bitch of the day

One of my favorite things to do is get together with girlfriends for an old-fashioned bitch session. It's as good as therapy: I get to vent about whatever is bugging me, and they do the same (kids, hubbies, weight, and in-laws seem to be popular topics). Then (maybe one or two glasses of rosé later), we give each other some great advice. So, here's your chance. I asked women to hit me up with their "bitch of the day," and in every chapter, I weigh in on how I think you can/should handle it. Of course, the decision is always yours—you have the power. But isn't it nice to know that someone is hearing you out and has your best interests at heart?

The sting of disappointment

I couldn't write a book about owning your power as a woman without talking about my recent devastation over the presidential election. No matter which side you're on, no matter your political position, we all have to agree on one thing: we did not elect the first woman president of the United States. We did not shatter the glass ceiling.

Disappointment shouldn't be something you just learn to accept and live with. You should evolve from it. Disappointment comes in all shapes and sizes. When things in life fail to meet my expectations, whether it's something small or a mammoth letdown, I feel sadness, anger, and despair, like someone has sucked all the air out of my lungs.

My friend, Dr. Robi Ludwig, author of *Your Best Age Is Now*, explains that the best way to deal with disappointment is to acknowledge it. "Yes, it's painful. Yes, it hurts, but it's also a natural part of life," she says. "Disappointment can humble us and shape us to be better human beings. If we learn from our disappointments, it can help us to navigate our lives in a way that makes us better, happier, stronger. The goal is always to use all of our painful experiences to help make us better people and better prepared for this thing called life."

So that's exactly what I do. I allow myself a few moments or even a few days to process it, and then I kick it to the curb. As a full-fledged bitch, you need to understand that disappointment is a major motivator. It spurs you onward and upward. It lights a fire under your butt and makes things a lot clearer. You see, disappointment and I go way back. When I was three years old, I knew my father was very sick. He would come home from work every day and throw up. Some days I would wait for him with a pot at the door. I wanted to help him, but I didn't realize how sick he truly was until my grandmother—who was the strongest woman I have ever known—told me. She took me to see my father at Sloan Kettering, where he was hooked up to several IVs.

On the way to the hospital, my grandmother explained to me that my dad was getting medicine to help him get better and stronger. She told me he was going to be okay. Yes, we were all upset that this happened to him. No, we didn't have any answers as to why. But it would be okay because we wouldn't accept the alternative.

I believed her. But I also came to understand that life is not fair—period. My friends' fathers were healthy and happy and could take them to the park or out for ice cream and go to their dance recitals. Mine couldn't, and I missed out on that. But I had no choice except to be brave for my mom. I wanted to be strong for her, and today, even at the age of forty-three, I think I still play that role.

However, there was an undercurrent of fear and worry surrounding our family that we didn't speak about. What if he didn't get better? What if he got worse? I thought it hundreds of times, but I didn't dare say it out loud—I didn't want to jinx it. I just wondered, why it was happening to *my* dad? Why not someone else's? The "whys" are a big part of disappointment; we demand a rational answer from an irrational world. Sometimes the rug is pulled out from under you and there is simply no explanation for it—or at least not one that we can know in this moment in time. That is disappointment in its simplest form.

After a year of chemo and radiation, the doctors announced that they felt confident my dad was in remission. My mom was as strong as one could be. I cannot remember a time when she complained, and I cannot remember her even shedding a tear in front of me. She took what life gave her and ran with it. She was my father's biggest supporter and cheerleader. She showed me how to handle life's curve balls—you knock them out of the park.

My dad went on to lead a good healthy life until he was in his early forties, when he was diagnosed with esophageal cancer. He was given six months to live. My mom, not one to be discouraged, found a treatment that stretched those six months into more than twenty years, even though he was not the strongest or healthiest during those additional years he was given. He passed away at age sixty-six.

People ask me all the time, "How do you cope?" You keep moving. You don't become paralyzed by disappointment. Honestly, in my effort to push forward, I did not take enough time to mourn properly. That is why going on a retreat was so emotionally empowering. I finally had a chance to let my emotions flow. I did a lot of crying, soul searching, and moving within those few days that I was by myself. It was something I needed to do for myself.

So, yes, when we failed to elect our first woman president I was dumfounded. But I didn't let it set me back for long. I have learned that you can't be a victim of your circumstance. You have to accept it and let it empower you. I always teach my kids that when one door closes, another one will open. You cannot live in fear or dread. We must live each day to the fullest.

My son, Ollie, is a huge fan of the play *Hamilton*, and we love to listen to the soundtrack. One lyric in particular, from the song "My Shot," strikes a chord with me: "Rise up! When you're living on your knees, you rise up!" That to me is how you cope with disappointment. You rise up until the next one knocks you to the ground, and then you rise up again, stronger and more determined than before. Following the election, I talked to a lot of women about disappointment—it was all people wanted to talk about.

Dr. Ludwig explains it well: "Figure out how to mourn your loss and then figure out, like a GPS system, how to re-navigate where you need to go when you find yourself off course. Sometimes we don't know why things happen, and we certainly don't have control over everything that happens to us. Disappointments are not the end of the road, but in fact, just a detour."

How a bitch handles disappointment

Get in touch with your emotions. It's okay to be pissed, sad, anxious, overwhelmed. Been there, done that. Let yourself feel what you need to feel and don't apologize for it. Break some dishes, bawl, throw a tantrum, hibernate, whatever works. Then, once your head is a little clearer, ask yourself what about this situation is making you feel this way. Were your expectations realistic (see below)? Were you making excuses for someone/something? Were you shutting your eyes to a situation and sugarcoating it to protect yourself? What made this disappointment so powerful, and how can you arm yourself against it in the future?

Manage your expectations. In a nutshell, expect virtually nothing from anyone, and no one will disappoint you. I'm not kidding; people can't hurt your feelings if you don't give them that power over you.

Don't take it personally. You have to tell yourself, *this isn't about me*. You didn't cause it to happen. You're not a magnet for bad things and bad people. Shit happens, plain and simple. Don't blame yourself or think that it's your fault. Disappointment can actually build character and confidence. Once you move past a disappointment, you can look back and be proud of the stronger, wiser person you became because of it.

Look on the bright side. By this, I mean find something (*anything*) positive that you can take away from this disappointment: a lesson learned, a truth garnered, a solution, or a compromise. You can't always control the situation, but you *can* control how you react to it. Bitches don't believe in negativity—we eat the stuff for breakfast.

If They Survived, So Can I . . .

These women looked disappointment in the eye and bulldozed over it. They inspire us all.

Jackie O: Her husband was assassinated right next to her. Instead of falling apart, she became a symbol of strength and grace for a grieving nation—not to mention a fashion icon.

Jennifer Hudson: Her mother, brother, and seven-year-old nephew were murdered by her eldest sister's estranged husband. Yet she found the strength to forgive their killer and started a children's charity in her nephew's name.

Jennifer Aniston: Brad dumped her for Angelina, but she has always retained her class, despite her life being displayed in the public eye. Now she is happily married to actor Justin Theroux.

Gwen Stefani: When divorcing Gavin Rossdale, she confided, "I really just wanted to be in bed crying and do what you do when your life falls apart." Instead, she channeled her emotion into her music and is dating Blake Shelton.

J. Lo: She's the queen of bouncing back from a breakup—a role model for us all! After splitting with both Ben Affleck

---

and Marc Anthony, she proved that she doesn't need a man to define her. The lady rocks on!

Katy Perry: When she split from Russell Brand, she chose not to cower. Instead, she put it into her concert documentary *Part of Me*. Take that!

Taylor Swift: The singer/songwriter is known for turning her splits with guys (perhaps you've heard of a few of them: John Mayer, Harry Styles, and Joe Jonas, just to name a few) into chart-topping pop songs. Any guy who dates her better beware . . . there's some future sheet music with your name on it.

Bitch of the Day

"I hate conflict. I just don't have the guts to stand up to people who put me down"

If you hate conflict, then that's all the more reason to tell someone (if the situation presents itself) to cease and desist. You're putting an end to the argument. You're literally shutting the door, declaring, "I'm done. This is over." Do you put a cap on the maple syrup bottle before it spills all over the place and makes a sticky mess? You bet you do. If someone is dissing you, or making unreasonable demands, you don't have to take it. You *shouldn't* take it. Personally, I would rip him/her a new one, but maybe you're not a woman of as many words. That's fine: keep it short and sweet. Spell it out: N-O.

STEP 2
GET YOUR SHIT TOGETHER

Fitz: "So, Abby's kind of a bitch."

Olivia Pope: "Don't say that! The words used to describe women! If she was a man you'd say she was 'formidable' or 'bold' or 'right.' "

—Scandal

You can't do everything and be everywhere, not unless the FDA suddenly approves a cloning treatment and Bliss Spa starts selling it (in which case, I'm first in line). On any given day, I feel like I'm the stretched and fraying rope in a never-ending game of a tug-of-war. My kids want this; my work needs that; my husband wants . . . Men are not meant to be multitasking; their minds just don't work that way. They can focus on one thing at a time, and everything else becomes chatter in the wind. I could tell my hubby to take the garbage out ten times in a row, and it will still be there in the morning. Why? Because he was busy watching the Mets game, and guys simply cannot take out the trash and fist-pump simultaneously. So, that leaves me (and only me) to cope with a mountain of to-dos that must get done. Is it fair? Of course not. No one said motherhood was fair.

I've considered going on strike several times, but then I'd have to explain to my kids why I was marching around our living room with a picket sign. Here's a better option—actually three options: prioritize, organize, and, most important, delegate. It takes a village—or in my case a large, cosmopolitan city—to raise a family. My friend Aliza Licht, founder and president of Leave Your Mark LLC, knows that motherhood is like running a business. "Being a mother is like being a CEO," she says. "You have to know how to delegate without guilt. You need to be both fearless and shameless in asking for what you need. You have to empower your team to achieve the most success. A happy family runs like a world-class company. It takes love, passion, dedication, and the power of collaboration. No one achieves anything great alone."

Take my kids . . . please!

I hate to put the blame on the fruit of my womb, but frankly, they ain't easy. I have a teenager, a preteen, and a toddler. Someone up there must be getting a good chuckle out of this. My kids are at three distinct stages of development, each requiring very different and specific things. What's the one thing they have in common? They all think mommy is the key to survival. Don't get me wrong; I love to be needed. But do they have to need me so much and so often? It's overwhelming, and with three to juggle, it's a given that one or two of them will fall by the wayside. Have I accidentally handed my thirteen-year-old a sippy cup of apple juice at breakfast? Um, yeah. Have I sworn like a truck driver in front of my two-year-old? Guilty as charged. I love my kids, but there are days I just can't take them. That's when it's time to pass them off on friends and family . . . no apologies needed.

To grandmother's house we go. They want to spoil the little darlings rotten—let them. I mean it: allow your parents or in-laws to take over and do whatever they want, however they want, as long as they keep your offspring out of your hair. If they want to serve them soda and ice cream for breakfast, I'm cool with it. Stay up all night watching TV? Be my guest! Let your children think Gram and Gramps are way more fun than you are (they'll want to go back next week!). And for God's sake, resist the urge to micromanage. If you undermine them, they will not be willing to take the baton the next time you need to pass it. Don't send a detailed list or time schedule. Just pack 'em up and ship 'em out.

You will want to show gratitude when you pick up your brood. A polite thank-you will do, no need to grovel. And, if they wrecked the furniture or trashed the place, offer some cold, hard cash to cover the damages. However, they won't accept it, I promise you. Why? Because you have given them the greatest gift in the world: grandchildren. They can dote on them and play with them, but they don't have to keep them forever. They're your problem. Plus, it reminds them of their youth and vitality and reinforces their significance in your life. They love it, truly.

I remember the first time I pawned my kid off on my parents. I felt bad. I felt like I was passing the buck, but it was our wedding anniversary, and we had planned a trip to Jamaica for a few days to celebrate. My son was just six months old at the time, and I was worried my mom and dad couldn't handle it. In their day, diapers didn't come with Velcro. But when I picked up my baby boy, my mom wouldn't let go of him. I literally had to pry her fingers off his chubby little body, and I thought I saw her well up. I resisted the urge to say, "You want him? Keep him!" Instead, I promised, "See you soon, Nanadoll!" The next day, my phone rang with an offer I couldn't refuse: "When can I babysit my grandson again?" Eureka, I'd struck gold!

Playdate payback. You know all those times you cheerfully took some munchkin off her desperate mom's hands for an endless afternoon? Allowed yourself to be saddled with a slew of kids so a group of moms could hit up the Hermès sample sale? Yes, you're *that* mom—the one who always volunteers for school trips and is elected class parent every freakin' year because no one else wants the job. You think other moms are in awe of your dedication, but truly they look at you and see a beast of burden. They dump on you because they know you're holding your arms out, waiting for it. Even the nannies know your name and hand over their charges to your safekeeping—they want the time off, too!

I was horrified when I realized I had become this person. It happened somewhere between the sandbox and soccer practice—a smiling mother shook my hand and handed me her kid for safekeeping. I remember my son was around a year old, and a mom I barely knew cornered me to vent: "We have a reservation at this hot restaurant that's impossible to get into, but I can't find a sitter!" She looked at me with such hope in her eyes that I caved instantly: "Yeah, sure, I'll watch your kid for a few hours."

Well, those few hours turned into an entire night. She came back at 1:00 a.m., seven hours after she dropped him on my doorstep, and she didn't check in once to see how he was doing. I was fed up and frazzled. I had Elmo on replay for four hours! "Oh, Lyss, you are the best!" she said before I could voice my protest.

It took a mere twenty-four hours for the word to get out: Lyss is running free daycare! The vultures circled: "Lyss, would you mind . . . " Hell yeah, I minded. But I couldn't say it; I was too polite. Or maybe I wanted to give everyone the impression that I was some kind of Super Mom. Stupid. I was stupid. I had enough kids of my own; I certainly didn't need to take care of someone else's. But it took becoming a bitch to make me see the light. I'd been used and abused for years, and it was payback time.

One day, I decided to *tell,* not ask, another mom that my son was going home with her child after school. No apologies; her kid had been at my apartment for the previous twelve Thursdays. "Ollie wants to hang with you guys today," I stated. Her jaw hit the ground—where did this new assertive Lyss come from? I could see her mind racing: does this mean no more afternoons off for me? It was magical, one of my greatest moments in bitch history. I took back control. I won! Not only did she take my son that day, but for the next four consecutive Thursdays as well. I had a month of freedom, peace, and joy—utter Lyss bliss. This, my friend, is how it's done.

1. **Do not feel guilty**. I want you to understand that you are not asking a favor of your fellow parents; you are owed this. You've served your time. Don't beg, plead, or whimper. Simply state the facts: "Johnny is going to your house after school today." *Finito.* Don't punctuate that statement with a question mark; say it like you mean it. Like there is no other option. Does anyone give you an option? Didn't think so.

2. **Drop the bomb**. I also don't believe in several days' notice (allows them to think up an excuse or fake an illness). The day before will do just fine, and if the mom of your choice already has a playdate planned, I say the more the merrier: "Great! Ollie would love to join the fun!" Don't allow her to wriggle out of this. If she claims her son has strep, I wanna see a note from the pediatrician. If you give her an out, she'll take it.

3. **Never offer to reciprocate.** Bitches don't barter. Look at it this way: your kid will entertain hers for a few hours so she doesn't have to. She should be thanking you. If you feel a tinge of remorse, send your son with money for the ice cream truck and tell him to buy one for his buddy. And toss that mom a Creamsicle while you're at it. If she's like you, she probably hasn't eaten all day.

4. **Bribe your babysitter.** Throw money at the problem, especially if the problem is your kids are driving you to drink. Most babysitters can be bought with overtime pay. Wave the words "Time and a half" in front of them and see what happens. I had one lovely nanny who would sell her soul for a Starbucks gift card. All I had to do was bring her back a venti Frappuccino, and she would graciously add a few more hours to her day so I could get work done. A friend of mine could get more hours every morning out of her baby nurse if she had a bagel and lox waiting for her. Everyone has a price.

   If your hubby complains about the cost (bribes don't come cheap), remind him that no kids for the weekend equals more sex for him. I guarantee this will shut him up real fast. There's something very dirty about paying for sex, even if it is with his own wife. If you don't have funds to spare, offer your sitter the clothes off your back, literally. I know an Upper East Side mom who handed her nanny a bag filled with cast-offs from her closet, and the woman was more than happy to watch the kids on her day off.

   A word to the wise: some sitters think they have you over a barrel. You need them, so they assume they have the upper hand and can make all kinds of crazy demands and get away with it. Not in this bitch's book. Here's the thing: there is an entire bulletin board in my laundry room filled with names and numbers of women willing to work for me. No one is irreplaceable, but remember who's boss here: you are. I'm not saying disrespect a hardworking sitter, someone who is doing a wonderful job and loves your children like her own. Just don't let anyone take an Uber home if they live two blocks away or order in filet mignon for lunch. If the subway and a Subway sandwich is good enough for me, it's good enough for them.

5. **Spousal support.** Your husband needs to understand that giving you a few hours off while he watches the kids does not constitute choreplay. It's his damn job; he signed up for it when he knocked you up. He should offer, not have to be asked, and he should assume responsibility for anyone under the age of eighteen who happens to be living under your roof—not pass it off to you.

A lot of men (let's be honest, most of them) view taking care of the kids as a huge favor they're doing for you. Hello? They're his kids, too. When my kids pick their noses and belch loudly in public, they're more my husband's than mine. For a long time, I would delicately ask my hubby, "Would you mind staying with the boys while I run out for a few minutes?" I was literally asking his permission to go grocery shopping without a BabyBjörn strapped to my bosom. He'd hem and haw, then finally give in oh so magnanimously: "Sure, Honey! I'll do it for you." Which would leave me wanting to sarcastically respond: "Gee, HoneyBee, thanks. Thanks a helluva lot! You rock! How did I ever get so lucky?"

Time to change the 'tude that your hubby is harboring. This will take some effort. You're not gonna link arms with him and start singing, "We're All In This Together" from the finale of *High School Musical* (which, I guarantee, he has never watched, because why would he?). He will resist; he will fight back like his life depends on it. He will grit his teeth and whine and complain, but you will turn a deaf ear. You are going to dole it out, dish it up, and dictate what needs to be done and when. Start by making a list of all the things required in the next twenty-four hours to keep your children happy, healthy, and not swinging from the chandelier. You'll handle the Mommy & Me ballet class (you are Mommy, so that's a tough one to pass off). But he can do dentist appointments, basketball practice, even a quick run to Costco for diapers. He can and he will, without a grumble. Why? Because if he doesn't take out that mile-long sausage link in the diaper genie, you're not doing it. That's right, bub, this is what "I mean business" looks and smells like (a lot like poo).

At first, he won't know what hit him, but slowly and surely he will get with the program. Mine did. And he liked it. He felt needed, appreciated, loved by his kids. He felt accomplished! Yes, gentlemen, you too can learn to sterilize bottles in the microwave and help your son with his prealgebra homework. As for me, I actually had a few minutes to myself, thank you very much—and I never had to empty the damn Diaper Genie again. Mission accomplished.

Keepin' track

I did not start out as the most organized person on the planet. My bag used to be a bottomless junk heap, filled with random receipts, crayons, spare change, and a few stray Tic Tacs. Each kid only added to the chaos: now I had Pokémon cards and Shopkins to schlepp around, too. One day while I was out having lunch with my girlfriend, sans kids, I accidentally dropped my tote on the floor and was mortified when I saw all the crap that spilled out of it. So, that's where that wad of gum in Ollie's mouth yesterday wound up! I went home, dumped it all out on a table, and began to weed through it, deciding what I need and don't need to have in my bag on a daily basis. A bitch's bag is always prepared yet pared down to be effective, efficient, and empowering. Here are my must-haves:

1. **My phone.** I literally don't go anywhere—not even to the bathroom—without it. Besides keeping track of my schedule, my

contacts, my to-do lists, playlists for the gym, you name it, I load it up with kid-friendly apps, too. In a pinch, it acts as a pacifier for a screaming toddler. I just whip it out and open the "Feed Maxi" app on my iPhone . . . and suddenly the waterworks stop.

2. **A portable charger.** Preferably, it should be a lightweight one with enough power to charge you two or three times, or one that doubles as a phone case (I like the mophie). Make sure you charge the charger, or it won't do you a bit of good. I will also tuck a spare lightning cord and plug in my purse in case I'm somewhere with an outlet and can juice up.

3. **Pen and paper.** I know, so old-school, but you never know when you might need to take a note or hand your child something to scribble on. I also carry a Filofax planner (remember those from the nineties?) as backup. If my phone crashes, I still have my schedule and grocery list in hand.

4. **Feminine hygiene products**. At my age, nothing is a sure thing anymore, including my cycle. You never know, so be prepared.

5. **Emergency phone numbers.** A friend of mine printed out a credit card-size version of her list, had it laminated, and tucks it into her wallet. Pediatrician, babysitter, twenty-four-hour pharmacy, school nurse, liquor store that delivers . . . you get my drift.

6. **Snacks.** Not just for the kids, for me—when my blood sugar is plummeting because I haven't eaten in hours. I like a handful of almonds or dried mango, just a little something that will take the edge off and keep me from passing out. It's also a great idea to carry a bottle of water (something refillable, like a S'well bottle) so you can hydrate while you hustle through your day.

7. **Mini first aid kit.** A few Band-Aids and some Neosporin Neo To Go will do the trick. If my kid scrapes his knee, Dr. Mom has just what he needs to make it all better.

8. **Wipes and tissues.** You never want to leave the house without something to mop up blood, spit-up, a runny nose, etc.

9. **Swiss pocketknife.** I actually own a pink one that is attached to my keychain so I always have it. It has a nail file, tweezer, scissors, and a little blade in a neat, pretty, little package. It makes me feel very MacGyver.

10. **Cold, hard cash.** At least $20 and some spare change along with your arsenal of credit cards and instant-pay apps on your phone. I got in a cab the other day and the credit machine was out of order. Can you imagine? I was happy that I had $10 buried in my bag to pay the driver.

11. **Hand sanitizer.** I never leave home without a bottle of Purell in my purse. Why? Because if there is a germ to be found, my toddler will find it, touch it, and put it in her mouth. Or worse, wipe it on me. If you can't wash your hands in a bathroom, it's the next best thing—at least that's what I like to tell myself.

12. **Glasses.** Driving glasses, reading glasses, just-so-I-don't-walk-into-walls glasses, sunglasses. It's worth splurging on a second pair at LensCrafters just so you can have them in your purse.

Forget me not: how to keep track of your life and your kids' lives

I have to be perfectly honest here: my job title is really "Stern family personal assistant." There is nothing that gets planned, plotted, or purchased without me. I am the person who makes reservations, confirms pediatrician appointments, and figures out the quickest route on Waze. If there is an activity to be arranged, a party to go to, a haircut to be scheduled, the buck stops here. I am the keeper of all lists and calendars, and my husband will scratch his head and ask me for a recap every night: "What's on the agenda tomorrow?" It used to drive me insane, until I got super-organized, thanks to Barbara Reich, a professional organizer and author of *Secrets of an Organized Mom*.

"The reason to be organized is it eliminates stress—and being a mom is stressful enough," Reich explains. "Everything costs you more in terms of time, money, and stress when you're not organized." Here are her top five tips for keeping control of a million details without losing your marbles:

1. **Label everything**. If you don't, you can't hold people accountable for where things belong. You know that pile of chargers you have in the drawer? Label each one: for the phone, for the iPad, for the e-reader, for the camera. You'll never waste time looking for the right charger again.

2. **Make maintenance a priority**. Spend ten minutes at the end of every day restoring order. Put the toys back in the toybox; pick up dirty laundry from the floor and place it in the hamper; get the dishes out of the sink and into the dishwasher. Tidy up now so tomorrow you're not waking up to a mountain of mess.

3. **Plan ahead.** Do it the night before. The backpacks are always ready to go, with homework inside them. The kids' clothes are laid out for school, and yours are laid out for work. Lunches are made and in the fridge, labeled with each kid's name.

4. **Delegate tasks**. Just realize that you have to be comfortable even if it's not done "right." Maybe your husband is the one who makes the travel arrangements. Your kids make their own beds; your little one can fill the dog's bowl with water. You're teaching them to be responsible—don't bark if it's not *exactly* how you would do it.

5. **Communicate with one another**. Have a family meeting on Sunday night so everyone knows what's coming up that week: "I have a science fair on Tuesday"; "I have a ballet recital Wednesday"; "It's grandpa's birthday Saturday." This way you'll know what you need—poster board, an extra pair of tights, and a birthday gift —to make sure things go smoothly throughout the week and you won't have to run out at the last minute trying to track down a pair of size 4T pink tights.

Get an App (so you can get a life)

There are a ton of apps out there; my personal fave is Cozi Family Organizer. Everyone can log on and take a look at the upcoming day, week, month, or even year. I refer to it constantly, and I print out the "week at a glance" and put it on the fridge so everyone is sure to see it. The point is, everyone is so married to their phones these days (including my thirteen-year-old) that a constant reminder in the palm of their hands keeps everyone in sync.

Digital declutter

It's not just about keeping a clean house; it's about making your email a no-mess zone as well.

- Delete all those emails that are three (or more) years old; you don't need them, so get rid of them. If you really can't hit the delete button, then put them into a folder with the year labeled, such as 2013–2014, or whatever dates they are from. No one's inbox should contain three hundred emails.
- Check your email at designated times during the day, not every five minutes. You're wasting your time and distracting yourself from other things that need to be tackled.
- When you open an email, do these three things: read it, respond if necessary, then delete or file it.
- People will save emails as a visual reminder to do things—don't use it as a cue. Keep a separate to-do list and file that email away.
- Make sure you change the subject line to reflect what the email is about. An email chain can make you crazy. You send your hubby an email with the subject line "Dinner Saturday Night," but eventually it ends up being a discussion about taking your son to the orthodontist. If you ever have to dig up the details of the appointment, you won't know to look for it in an email you think is about the new Italian eatery in the hood.

Bitch of the Day

"My kids always forget to text me where they're going, and it makes me a basket case."

Let me tell you how my friend resolved this issue. Her thirteen-year-old daughter had a bad habit of "forgetting" to text or call her when she got to a friend's house after school. This poor mom was always having to chase her daughter down to make sure she was okay. One day, the daughter didn't respond to texts or calls from her mom (she was too busy). So, my friend decided it was time to teach her a lesson. She went on "Find My iPhone" and sounded her daughter's cell phone alarm. A shrill, piercing tone suddenly rang through 16 Handles, the local frozen yogurt shop, where a group of eighth graders were hanging out. Boy, did that kid pick up the phone fast! She was mortified, but she learned the lesson: call your mother or she will sound the alarm!

My advice to you is to be as specific as you can with your kids. Tell them, "I expect to hear from you, and if I don't, there will be consequences (e.g., the iPhone alarm or they won't be allowed to go out with friends for a week)." If they don't fulfill their end of the bargain, they lose any freedom or privileges they might have had. This is about building trust. Assure them that every time they do what you ask, you will become more comfortable and less clingy. If that doesn't work, I say superglue them to a chair at home so they don't give you anymore agita.

STEP 3
From Flab to Fab

"I like my body so much better after I had kids. Is that a crazy thing to say? I'm more womanly. I feel sexier."

—*Reese Witherspoon*

Some people have "Ah-ha!" moments. I have "WTF?" ones. Not long ago, I ran into a friend of mine I had not seen in a while on the street.

"Lyss!" she said, hugging me. "You look great!"

I smiled and thanked her. It was nice to hear, since I had no makeup on and was wearing the same Wonder Woman T-shirt for the third day in a row. Then she continued, "So, when are you due?"

My heart literally stopped beating. Due? As in pregnant? Did I look like I had a bun in the oven? Did I look *that big?*

"I had a baby two years ago," I told her through gritted teeth. "I'm not pregnant. I'm just fat."

Girlfriend backpedaled big-time. "Oh! You did? How wonderful! Good for you! Tootles!" Then she ran away before I could punch her in the face.

All the way home, I refused to look at my reflection in store windows. I felt awful. Is that how people really saw me? I went home, stripped down to my undies, and forced myself to take a good, hard look in the mirror. It wasn't pretty—my belly was bloated, and my ass looked huge. I had to admit my friend was kind of right, but I had a hunch where and when things had gone terribly wrong. I had let the stress of running my own business get to me, and I tried to calm that stress storm and lack of energy with comfort food. I felt depleted. Enough was enough; this bitch was getting her body back!

The first step in my plan was to banish any and all excuses, and I am the queen of excuses. They would go something like this: "I can't exercise today because . . .

- I'm too tired.
- I'm too busy.
- I'm too cold.
- I'm too hot.
- I have a headache.
- I have to be at a PTA meeting.
- I have four hours of *The Bachelorette* waiting for me on the DVR.

So, I made myself a promise that there would be no more reasons why I couldn't get in *some* form of physical activity at least twenty minutes a day—even if it killed me.

I had a long talk with my husband that evening. I explained that I needed to make serious life changes. I was joining Flywheel Sports, an indoor cycling studio, and Exhale fitness studio, and I was going to be eating healthier and cleaner. From now on the apartment would be stocked with healthy snacks, not just for the children, but for myself and for him as well. If I couldn't eat Ben & Jerry's, Oreos, or Doritos, neither could he. "I don't want to be tempted," I explained. "I'm weak. If you give Lyss a cookie, she will eat the entire box." He nodded and was 100 percent supportive, so the next day I jumped in with both feet and hit my very first spin class. I came out dripping sweat and legs trembling, but entirely empowered. I was doing something *for me.* It felt freakin' awesome.

Slowly and surely, the weight started to come off. I won't lie and say it melted away. There were days, even weeks, when it stubbornly clung to my body for dear life. My plateau was more like Mount Everest. But, eventually, I won the battle with the bulge. I lost twenty pounds and a few sizes. I still have a way to go, but that's okay: Rome wasn't built in a day, and neither were buns of steel. The point is, I am doing it. I took back control. I am changing what I have the power to change and covering the rest with Spanx!

I wish I could tell you that I don't miss sugar, but I do. I miss it a lot. Especially when I'm PMSing, I dream about it. But since my "transformation," I now have just a handful of Swedish Fish instead of the entire bag, and the same goes for my sour peach gummies. Now whenever a sugar craving hits, I drink fresh-pressed watermelon juice; it's sweet and keeps me hydrated. Once a week, I allow myself a Häagen-Dazs mint chip Dazzler. *Real Housewife of New York City* Kelly Killoren Bensimon once told me that she eats clean six days out of the week and one day is earmarked as her cheat day. It makes perfect sense to me: if you don't feel deprived, you won't be tempted to binge on bad stuff. Just knowing I have one day to eat pizza, pancakes, french fries, whatever my heart desires, helps me be good the rest of the week. But the one thing I simply cannot live without is a glass of rosé once a day. It's worth every calorie and keeps me sane. I say pick your poison. I'd rather eat like a rabbit all day so I can have my rosé at night.

These days, I am feeling much stronger and healthier both mentally and physically—the best I've felt in the twelve years since I had my first kid—but I'm also realistic. I know I will never be the size I was when I was single, and I'm okay with it. No, you can't bounce a quarter off my ass—so what? When did being a double-digit size become a stigma? There's a lot of judging and body shaming that goes on amongst the mommy set, and I don't think it's fair. Don't make fun of my bat wings unless you know what I've been through. Any fat on this body is armor! This is where your bitch attitude needs to take over; do not let others make you feel bad about yourself. Stop comparing. There will always be some mom who was blessed with (or paid for) a Victoria's Secret body. That doesn't make her better than you; it makes her skinnier, with bigger, not-so-bouncy boobs and a tight ass. (I'm trying hard not to hate here!) You get my drift. It's easy to find a million reasons to practice self-loathing, but bitches don't belittle themselves. You are taking positive steps and making healthy choices—that's enough of a reason to hold your head up high. Hopefully your boobs will take the hint and head in the same direction!

There are certain things I can live with when it comes to my body, and some I can't. It's a bitch's prerogative. I'm okay with never again running around the beach in a string bikini like I did in high school (oh, those were the days!). Instead, I have mastered the art of the flowy cover-up—and I let my kids bury my thighs in the sand. What I'm not cool with is people thinking I'm carrying twins, or having to retouch my double chins in selfies. So I work on those things. I make a conscious effort to eat less crap and move more. It's that simple: take charge of your body. Practice a lean, mean mentality, and the physical will follow.

Eating on the run

I feel like I never actually sit down for a meal—it's a rarity. I actually have to make a grand announcement in my home: "It's dinner and everyone—including me—is sitting down at this table." I'm lucky if it lasts ten minutes and I don't have to get up ten times to hand my kids the ketchup, pour more apple juice, or get a fork to replace the one someone dropped. Mornings are the hardest: there is always a hard-boiled egg or a glass of juice in my hand as I run out the door. I have learned to multitask this part of my life as well: eat and sprint at the same time. But that's a far cry from the old days when I would literally shove a bagel or a candy bar in my mouth. In a pinch, I would steal some of my daughter's Cheerios. This was no way to live, and no way to eat. Nutritionist Keri Glassman taught me that there are ways to snack smart, even if you have only seconds to fuel up.

Smart snacks to eat on the run

- Individual packet of nut butter (such as almond or peanut) with an apple.
- Popcorn (choose a non-GMO brand that comes prepackaged in a single-portion size) and eight to fifteen nuts, such as almonds, walnuts, or pecans (portion them out ahead of time).
- Four to six ounces of full-fat Greek yogurt topped with a dash of cinnamon and/or eight to fifteen nuts, such as almonds, walnuts, or pecans (portion them out ahead of time).

- Lettuce wrap: use a leaf of lettuce as the wrap, and spread with mustard, then add a slice of turkey, carrot slices, and roll up.
- Hummus (buy single-serving containers or portion on own) sprinkled with hemp seeds, and then dip slices of cucumber.
- EPIC protein bar—These are a whole new way to get protein into your diet, and they'll easily go wherever the day takes you (stash one in your bag). For all you paleo and gluten-free peeps, this is a home run. Made with grass-fed bison, one bar provides eleven grams of protein and will most definitely keep you satisfied until dinnertime.
- Dried chickpeas—Can you say protein, fiber, antioxidants, and crunch? OK, don't say it, just eat them. The Good Bean brand comes in both sweet and savory flavors, so all of your cravings are covered.

Why water is important

I know, I know—it's tasteless and a lot less sexy than a caramel macchiato. But water is the key to weight loss. It eliminates toxins (all the crap you've managed to accrue in your body) and keeps you hydrated. Here's a fun fact: the process of burning calories requires an adequate supply of water in order to function efficiently, and water helps the body metabolize and burn fat.

Benefits of Drinking Water

According to Keri, drinking water is a win–win for your body. It . . .

- helps you eat less at meals
- improves your mood
- makes your skin glow
- helps you lose and maintain weight
- helps you feel more energized

So, if you want to drop pounds, you can't do it if you're parched. Keri explained that there are ways to "sneak" water into your daily life. Basically, you must be mindful of how much water you're drinking. If an hour has gone by without a sip, it's too long. I try not to put a number on it, like "I'm going to drink sixty-four ounces of water today." That's just not practical, and it stresses me out. Instead, find ways to work it in that are slightly more appealing than guzzling down your average bottle of H2O:

- Make drinking water indulgent and different—add a little cinnamon, clove, and cardamom for an exotic flavor.
- Keep a pitcher of water with lemon and mint in your fridge at all times. For real, it tastes like an alcohol-free mojito! You'll want to keep sipping.
- Add pieces of frozen fruit to your glass or bottle of water. Try raspberries, strawberries, or mango. YUM!
- Eat foods that contain a high volume of water. Foods like cucumber (97 percent), radishes (95 percent), celery (95 percent), and watermelon (91 percent) are all high in water and contribute to your daily water intake sans the water glass.
- Get excited about it. Buy yourself a new twenty-five-ounce water bottle (S'well makes really cool, colorful ones that stay cold for hours). Bring it everywhere with you, and sipping water throughout the day will quickly become a good habit.

The bitchy mama diet

I want food, real food, that tastes good. That was my one caveat when I asked Keri to put together a meal plan for me. I also wanted choices, because bitches get bored easily. I cannot eat the same breakfast three days in a row; I need variety. Finally, there had to be things that my family would eat—like taco night—because I'm not running a restaurant. I asked for quick, simple, healthy, and delish, and she delivered. Her website (www.nutritouslife.com) is filled with even more great options for moms on a mission to get their bods back.

The Bitch Recipe Box

Breakfast:

- Slice of sprouted grain toast with one-third avocado, mashed. Add a dash of sea salt and pepper and top with a slice of tomato. For a little heartier breakfast, add a sliced hard-boiled egg.
- Six ounces of full-fat Greek yogurt with a sprinkle of cinnamon and topped with fresh or frozen berries. Add one tablespoon of sliced almonds. I serve this to my boys as a "breakfast sundae," and they love it.
- Half cup of steel-cut oatmeal with two teaspoons of almond or peanut butter mixed in. Top with one small or one-half of a large banana, sliced.

Avocado-Banana Smoothie

Don't be fooled by the fact that it's green—this tastes amazing and fills you up for hours.

Servings: 1   Prep Time: 5 minutes

Ingredients:

1 cup almond milk, unsweetened
1 small banana, frozen
1 tablespoon peanut butter or almond butter
½ small avocado
1 handful spinach, raw
1 scoop Life's Abundance Vanilla Protein Powder

Directions:

Place all ingredients into a Vitamix or other blender and blend until it reaches the desired thickness.

Veggie and Cheddar Mini Quiche

Double the recipe so you can make this ahead and store in fridge for weekday morning reheating!

Servings: 6   Prep Time: 10 minutes + cooking time

Ingredients:

1 tablespoon + 2 teaspoons wheat germ
1 tablespoon ground flaxseed
2 omega-3-enriched eggs
2 egg whites
2 tablespoons whole milk
½ cup low-fat cottage cheese
⅛ teaspoon garlic powder
¼ teaspoon fresh-ground black pepper
¼ teaspoon fresh tarragon, finely chopped
¼ cup cheddar cheese, shredded
1 cup broccoli, cooked and chopped
½ cup mushrooms, chopped
Parmesan cheese, optional

Directions:

1. Preheat the oven to 350°F. Coat a 6-cup nonstick muffin pan with cooking spray.
2. Combine the wheat germ and flaxseed in a small bowl. Add 1 heaping teaspoon of the mixture to each muffin cup, spreading to coat the bottoms evenly.
3. Whisk together the eggs, egg whites, milk, and cottage cheese in a bowl.
4. Add the garlic powder, black pepper, tarragon, and cheddar cheese, then whisk until combined.
5. Stir in the broccoli and mushrooms, then divide the mixture among the muffin cups, using ¼ cup measures.

6. Place the pan on the middle rack of the oven and bake for 30 to 35 minutes or until the mini quiches are lightly browned on top and a knife inserted in the center comes out clean.
7. Place the pan on a wire rack and allow the quiches to cool for 5 to 10 minutes. Using a large knife, loosen the edges from the sides of the pan and remove the mini quiches. If desired, sprinkle with Parmesan cheese and serve.

Lunch:

- Open-faced sammy. Spread some Dijon mustard on a slice of Ezekiel bread, then add 3–4 slices sliced of roasted turkey breast, 1 tomato slice, and ¼ avocado, and top with alfalfa sprouts. Toss 1 cup of artichoke hearts on top for some added filling fiber, then squeeze on lemon juice. Add a cup of blueberries on the side.
- Everything-but-the-kitchen-sink sampler plate. Start with fresh, raw veggies, such as carrots and peppers. Add two tablespoons of hummus or guacamole; a few slices of roasted chicken, turkey, ham, or chicken sausage; and a sliced peach or tangerine.
- Lettuce-free chopped salad. Cut up a cucumber, carrots, celery, radishes, and red peppers (make a big portion and store in the fridge) When ready to eat, top with 4 to 6 ounces of tuna or chickpeas and 1 tablespoon of feta, then drizzle with balsamic or red wine vinegar. Add dried oregano for an antioxidant and flavor boost.

Green Goddess Edamame Salad and Dressing

Okay, you had me at "goddess." This is a great choice when you're tired of the same ol' salad.

Servings: 2   Prep Time: 15–20 minutes

Ingredients:

Dressing:

2 tablespoons fat-free plain yogurt

1 tablespoon raw pistachios, shelled and finely chopped

1 tablespoon steeped green tea, cooled to room temperature

1 tablespoon green onion, thinly sliced

1 teaspoon parsley, finely chopped

1 teaspoon red wine vinegar

½ teaspoon minced garlic

Salt and fresh-ground black pepper

Salad:

¾ cup frozen edamame, shelled

½ cup celery, thinly sliced

⅓ cup artichoke hearts, chopped and marinated

¼ cup radishes, thinly sliced

Directions:

1. To make the dressing: Combine the yogurt, pistachios, tea, onion, parsley, vinegar, and garlic in a small bowl. Season to taste with salt and pepper. Set aside.
2. To make the salad: Defrost the edamame in the microwave, according to the package directions. Let it cool to room temperature.
3. Toss the edamame, celery, artichoke hearts, and radishes with the dressing and serve.

Dinner:

- Broiled salmon. Top the salmon with Dijon and soy sauce then broil. Serve with broccoli.
- Shrimp stir-fry. Always keep frozen shrimp on hand to stir-fry (with 2 teaspoons coconut oil). Stir-fry the shrimp

with a mixture of veggies, such as red peppers, snow peas, and mushrooms. Serve over ½ cup quinoa or brown rice. Another option: toss shrimp with marinara sauce and serve over steamed broccoli. Top with 1 tablespoon Parmesan cheese.

- Tasty tacos. Tacos make everyone at home happy and are the perfect fast, flavorful option when you're bored of the same old grilled chicken. Use grass-fed ground beef, or kidney and black beans for a vegetarian option. Serve with corn tortillas or whole wheat tortillas (no fried chips or shells necessary!). Or, skip the tortillas altogether and serve over chopped romaine. Get creative with veggies to top the tacos with. Try sliced red and yellow peppers, mushrooms, tomatoes, zucchini; almost any veggies you have on hand will work. Then, skip the cheese and serve with guacamole and salsa, and Greek yogurt in place of sour cream. Sriracha always works for extra spice.

Greek Yogurt-Marinated Chicken

I got tired of my hubby and kids whining, "Chicken? Again?" This dish has tons of flavor, and I can always cut it up over a salad for me and serve it to them as DIY fajitas in a wrap with all the fixin's (cheese, guacamole, veggies) on the side. Tell my middle son, Ollie, that he can "make" his own dinner, and he's happy.

Servings: 6–8   Prep Time: 10 minutes

Ingredients:

1 cup low-fat Greek yogurt
1 tablespoon olive oil
1 teaspoon chili powder
1 garlic clove, minced
Salt and pepper, to taste
2 pounds chicken breasts

Directions:

1. Whisk together the yogurt, olive oil, chili powder, garlic, salt, and pepper in a bowl.
2. Place the chicken in a container, then pour the marinade over the top. Cover and let sit in the refrigerator overnight.
3. When you're ready to prepare the chicken, preheat the grill or prepare a medium-size sauté pan with a light coat of olive oil and place over medium-high heat on the stove.
4. Remove the chicken from the marinade and season with additional salt and pepper to taste.
5. Brush the hot grill grates lightly with oil and grill the chicken over medium heat. If cooking on the stove, lay the chicken in the prepared pan and cook over medium-high heat, flipping halfway through. For either method, cook until the chicken reaches an internal temperature of 165°F.

Dessert

- Almond vanilla popsicles. Indulge in a tasty frozen treat. Combine 1 cup unsweetened almond milk, 1 teaspoon vanilla extract, 1 tablespoon honey, and ⅛ cup of slivered almonds in a blender until smooth. Pour into popsicle molds. Insert wooden sticks once they are semifirm. Freeze until they are completely frozen.
- Peanut butter berry yogurt. A healthy twist on a childhood favorite. Combine ¾ cup low-fat Greek yogurt with 1 tablespoon natural peanut butter. Top with ½ cup fresh berries.

Fudgy Chocolate Chickpea Brownies

Keri's healthier version of my kids' fave homemade sweet treat is a huge hit. Don't tell them it has chickpeas in it for protein!
Servings: 12
Prep time: 10 minutes + baking time

Ingredients:

1¼ cups 70% cacao chocolate chips
4 eggs
1 19-ounce can chickpeas/garbanzo beans, drained and rinsed
¾ cup turbinado sugar
½ teaspoon baking powder
Powdered sugar and cinnamon or cocoa powder for dusting (2:1 ratio)

Directions:

1. Preheat the oven to 350°F and lightly coat a 9-inch baking pan with cooking spray.
2. Place the chocolate chips in an oven-safe bowl and melt them as the oven preheats. (Keep an eye on them and stir them often!)
3. Put the eggs and chickpeas in a food processor and combine them into a smooth mixture.
4. Add the sugar and baking powder and combine well.
5. Add the melted chocolate chips (use a spatula and not your finger to get it all in there).
6. Mix well and then transfer to the baking pan.
7. Bake for 40 minutes. A toothpick inserted in the middle should come out clean; if it doesn't, bake for a few more minutes.
8. Place the pan on a wire rack and allow the brownies to cool before turning them onto a serving plate.
9. Dust with the powdered sugar and cinnamon/cocoa mixture when the brownies are completely cooled. Cut into squares and serve.

Fill 'er up

My friend, diet guru Tanya Zuckerbrot, MS, RD, created the F-Factor Diet (http://ffactor.com) and wrote two best-selling books (*The F-Factor Diet: Discover the Secret to Permanent Weight Loss* and *The Miracle Carb Diet: Make Calories and Fat Disappear— with Fiber*). She also knows a thing or two about being a harried working mom—she has three kids. "It's important to be in control of our diets and to stay healthy and fit, because as mothers— whether working or stay-at-home—we often have to-do lists that are miles long. But your job description as a mom does not include eating the scraps of food leftover from your children's meals. You're not a garbage disposal. You're a dignified woman, treat yourself like one: leave scraps of chicken nuggets to the actual garbage disposal and serve yourself a real meal!" You said it, sister!

She also taught me the importance of integrating high-fiber foods into my daily diet, so I wasn't tempted to nibble (okay, pig out!) as the day went along and I felt myself waning. "Fiber is the secret nutrient for losing weight without hunger, as it helps eliminate the hunger pangs associated with dieting," Tanya explains. "Fiber is the zero-calorie, nondigestible part of a carbohydrate that adds bulk to food. When you follow a diet rich in fiber, you feel full after eating, so you'll generally eat less throughout the day." Most of us fall short on getting the recommended twenty-five grams a day, but, according to Tanya, there are so many good reasons to fill up on fiber:

- Fiber slows digestion and steadies blood sugar levels, which curbs sugar cravings and sustains energy.
- Fiber boosts metabolism. The human body can't digest fiber, but it attempts to, burning calories in the process.
- Fiber swells in the stomach, absorbing calories and fat from other foods in the meal before the body can absorb them.
- High-fiber foods satisfy hunger because they require more chewing, which prompts the secretion of saliva in the mouth

and gastric juices in the stomach that promote satiety by signaling the brain, "I'm full!"

- Studies have shown that diets high in fiber reduce the risk factors for cardiovascular disease, adult onset diabetes, hypertension, and certain forms of cancer including breast and colon cancer.

Foods rich in fiber

Tanya recommends you aim for seven or more grams of fiber at breakfast, lunch, and dinner, plus one to two snacks with three or more grams of fiber each. For starters, try some of these fiber-rich foods:

- Fresh strawberries, blackberries, raspberries, apricots, and figs all offer a sweet fiber boost. One cup of raspberries or a ½ cup of figs has 8 grams of fiber.
- Pomegranate seeds. Buy them already removed from the shell. A ½ cup has 4 grams of fiber and makes a great snack. You can also sprinkle them on top of yogurt, cereal, or oatmeal.
- Barley. Like rice, oatmeal, and quinoa, barley is a grain that puffs up as it cooks, meaning a little bit goes a long way toward keeping you full. Just 1 cup, cooked, has 6 grams of fiber. Can you say, "super side dish"?
- Artichokes. Just one steamed artichoke has 10 grams of fiber and is a natural detoxifier.
- Roasted acorn squash. One cup, cubed, packs 9 grams of fiber. You can serve it up mashed, seasoned with cinnamon or nutmeg, instead of potatoes.
- Avocado. I love these on everything from salads to sandwiches, and it provides 8 grams of fiber per ½ cup serving.
- Black beans. I used to think you only ate these at Mexican restaurants. Now I know that sneaking in a ½ cup into rice or quinoa loads you up with 15 grams of fiber.

The five in ten shape-up plan

I owe a lot to Elisabeth Halfpapp and Fred DeVito at Exhale for whipping my sorry ass back into shape. They are my gurus of barre exercise and even wrote a book about it (*Barre Fitness: Barre Exercises You Can Do Anywhere for Flexibility, Core Strength, and a Lean Body*). But not everyone has time or money to get into a gym or exercise studio. Never fear, all you need is 10 minutes a day at home and these five exercises to get your butt, abs, thighs, and arms looking leaner. Do them for 2 minutes each; you can even split them up if you don't have 10 consecutive minutes to spare. The important thing is to make them a habit—each and every day—and feel that burn.

The Table Top (lifts your butt)

- Come to the floor on your hands and knees: ensure that your wrists are under your shoulders and your knees are directly under your hips.
- Pull your abs in to support your lower back, then extend your left leg straight behind your left hip with the foot flexed.
- Raise your left leg hip-high, keeping your hips square to the floor and your right shin firmly tacked against the floor for support.
- Lift your left leg up an inch and hold for a count of ten. Release down an inch, then raise and hold. Repeat twenty times per set. Complete three sets.
- With your left leg still extended, bend your left knee, bringing your left heel toward your butt.
- Keeping the knee bent, lift your left leg up an inch and hold for a count of ten. Release down an inch, then lift and hold again. Repeat twenty times per set. Complete three sets.
- Repeat on the right leg.

Pelvic Lifts (tightens your butt)

- Lie on your back with your knees bent and feet flat on the floor, with your ankles under knees. Your feet should be hip width apart.
- Raise your butt up off the floor, pressing your hips up toward the ceiling.
- Pull your abs in to support your lower back and contract your glutes and hamstrings as you raise your hips.
- Lift your hips to their highest point and hold for a count of ten. Release down about 1 inch, then raise the hips again and hold. Repeat twenty times per set. Complete three sets.
- Touch your butt to the floor, then lift your hips as high as you can and hold for a count of ten. Allow your butt to touch the floor, then lift your hips again and hold. Repeat twenty times per set. Complete three sets.
- Lift your heels, bring your toes under your knees. Lift your hips to their highest point with small, quick lifts. Repeat twenty times per set. Complete three sets.

Forearm Plank (tones your tummy)

- Come to the floor and lie on your stomach. Lift your upper body by placing your forearms shoulder width apart, with your elbows directly under your shoulders. Keep your forearms parallel with your palms flat on the floor or move the hands together so you can interlace your fingers.
- Keeping your knees on the floor, lift your hips up to the same height as your shoulders.
- Pull in your abdominals and hold them in. Do not allow your breathing to move or release your abdominal brace. Breathe high up in the lungs instead of low in the belly.
- Hold this position for 30 to 60 seconds to start.
- If you feel strong enough and you aren't experiencing any discomfort in your lower back, straighten your legs while keeping your hips in line with your shoulders.

- Gradually increase your time until you can hold a straight leg plank, with your abdominals pulled in and lower back supported, for up to 2 minutes nonstop.

Single Leg Strengthener (firms up your thighs)

- Stand with your back against something stable (a heavy chair, countertop, wall, etc.) for support.
- Extend your left leg straight out in front of you, with the foot pointed, and lift the leg up as high as you can, with the goal being to get it hip high.
- Lift the leg up as high as it can go and hold for a count of ten. Then lower the leg slightly, lift again, and hold. Repeat twenty times per set. Complete three sets.
- Hold the last one for eight counts while raising your arms above your shoulders to balance.
- Repeat on the right side.

Supermom Push-ups (tones your arms and upper body)

- Come to the floor on your hands and knees, walk your knees back until your hips are down and flat on the floor.
- Place your hands a little wider than your shoulders, with your fingers pointing forward.
- Pull your abdominals in to support your lower back.
- Bend your elbows to lower your body toward the floor in a straight (plank-like) line. Straighten your elbows, pressing your body up away from the floor and back to the starting position.
- Do ten times per set. Complete three sets.
- Once you've mastered this exercise with bent knees, start doing it with your legs straight.

Bitch of the Day

I never have a minute to myself! Every time I try and nap, shower, or breathe, my kids whine or my husband finds something else for me to do. I feel like an indentured servant!

I get it—they're treating you like you belong downstairs on *Downton Abbey*. You run the house, and it runs you ragged. Girlfriend, you need to take action. I've actually locked myself in the bathroom on more than one occasion just to get a few minutes of peace and quiet (or do a crossword puzzle). Just as you carefully plan out your day to accommodate everyone else's needs, you need to schedule in some time for yourself. When was the last time you had a facial? A pedi? Got your teeth cleaned? You hear what I'm saying? You're entitled. Make the time for yourself because no one else will. And I highly recommend running away for a day or two. Whenever I go on a retreat or to a spa—even if it's only for twenty-four hours—I come back a new woman. If the hubby and kids protest, too bad. Mommy needs to recharge her batteries or she's going to be no good for anyone, including herself. Happy mom = happy kids.

STEP 4
BRING SEXY BACK

"I don't judge others. I say if you feel good with what you're doing, let your freak flag fly."

—Sarah Jessica Parker

I used to be chic, I swear. I hit every designer sample sale in New York City, always looked polished and put-together (or at least I thought so), and wore nothing less than four-inch stilettos, even on the subway. Carrie Bradshaw had nothin' on me! Then I had kids, and, well, you know how that story goes. Even SJP was photographed taking her twins to school wearing flip-flops and looking like she fell out of bed. It happens to the best of us—even style icons.

But most moms snap out of it once the 2:00 a.m. feedings subside. Me, not so much. The problem is that just when I thought my baby-rearing days were behind me, my daughter came along. It threw me for a loop, and my fashion sense took a beating as well. Right after Blakey was born, I would describe my style as "frumpy-dumpy," and I'm being kind. I rarely wore anything beyond yoga pants, sneakers, and the occasional baseball hat (to cover greasy, graying hair). At least, I told myself, you're out of your maternity clothes. To be honest, they would have been an improvement. I stopped shopping and reading fashion magazines—who has freakin' time when you have a newborn? I told myself I looked fine when people were mistaking me on the street for an Olsen twin (from their grunge phase) or a bag lady. Yeah, it was *that bad*.

So, when I hit reboot and became a bitch, I decided my outer appearance needed to match my inner fabulosity. Especially since I would soon be hosting my Fourth Annual DivaMoms Mom Mogul Breakfast and had to look halfway human for an audience of three hundred women. I remember wishing I had the money to hire a celebrity stylist to fix me; they can work wonders. Rumor has it that Kim Kardashian pays her stylist a million bucks to keep them on retainer, and I just want to say, "You go, girl!"

Since I had no personal stylist on the payroll, I descended on Lord & Taylor's, where I found a lovely (and free!) personal shopper to help me navigate the dress department. I had no idea what size I was, or even what style would look good on me. He put together a rack of options, but I was still overwhelmed. After texting selfies to several of my friends, I chose a simple, cream-colored sheath with a beaded neckline to draw the eye up (look at my face, not my belly bulge!). It skimmed my hips and waist without being too tight and fell just above the knee— perfection. Then I added a nude heel to lengthen my legs. It felt *sooo good*. I held my head high as I strutted around the store's dressing room. The bitch was on her way back.

Losing a few sizes was the incentive I needed to rethink my wardrobe and edit it (see below). When the credit card bills arrived and he started hyperventilating, I told my husband that I had no choice, everything was literally falling off me. It was either shop or risk flashing the elementary school security guard when I bent over. I invested in jeans—really great-fitting jeans— that make my ass and hips look good. My clothes are more fitted and tailored now, rather than baggy and shapeless. And, bonus, they're not stained. It's amazing how simple it really is. You don't need a lot of pieces, just a few staples that you can mix and match. You also need to abide by a few rules. Your clothes should . . .

- Fit flawlessly. If it bags, buckles, billows out—say buh-bye. When you feel fat, you tend to break out the tents and muumuus to cover it up. I can't begin to tell you how many pashmina shawls and ponchos I had for camouflage duty. But big clothes make you look bigger. If something doesn't fit you to perfection, find yourself a good tailor. It's worth every penny to have something custom-fit to your body. Rarely do I find a piece of clothing I can wear without altering it, even if it's just to take the waist in a tad or the hemline up an inch. Some stores will even do it for you for free (or a small fee) when you buy the item there.

- Feel good on your body. The material can't itch, poke, cling, or flash the world your lady parts. I saw a mom the other day at a trendy New York City lunch spot, dressed in a stunning chiffon blouse. Then I looked a little closer as she leaned forward over her lobster salad: her nipples were poking through the thin fabric ... *quelle horreur!* Save it for the boudoir, not Freds at Barneys!

- Celebrate you. I know you've heard people say this before, but confidence truly is a woman's best accessory. If I'm happy with what I'm wearing, I hold my head high. I hate when I hear moms saying, "I can't wear that! I'm a mother." So what? Does that mean you have to dress like June Cleaver? Bitches grab fashion by the balls. I don't care what others think of me; I care what I think of myself. You should feel the same. If something empowers and elevates you, then buy it and *truly* own it. You should never let anyone dictate what you wear—not a stylist, not your girlfriends, not a magazine. Style maven, author, and mom of twins, Sasha Charnin Morrison was named one of the Top 10 Most Powerful People in Fashion by *Radar* magazine, so she knows what she's talkin' about. Sasha said to me, "There's something about keeping up with everyone's perception of what you should be or need to be that has never interested me. My mother raised me to never give a rat's ass about what people thought about me. The people I used to worry about are now in prison, you know? You have to find strength within you. It's there. We all have it."

Ten things to toss because they scream "Frumpy Mom!"

Tiffany Keriakos, owner of Designer Revival, a New York City consignment shop, has helped me unload my closet on numerous occasions. Her rule is simple: for each new item you buy or add, get rid of one you don't wear. These items will not be missed:

1. **Sweat suits.** Unless you're actually wearing them to the gym, you don't need a collection of hoodies and track pants. I understand the whole "athleisure" movement, but most of those women

(Hello, Kate Hudson!) who rock it have six-pack abs and buns of steel. If you have neither at the moment, then I beg you, banish anything with a swoosh or a stripe from your everyday attire.

2. **Baggy T-shirts.** Shapeless ones, especially those that have spit-up stains and holes in them, just need to go. It killed me to get rid of my old Syracuse University tees, but they'd certainly seen better days. They do make great dust rags, though.

3. **Anything with horizontal stripes.** No grown woman should strive to look like Tigger or Waldo; the stripes just make you appear wider. Unless you are stick-thin or heading to a costume party, please fuggedaboutit.

4. **Long cardigans.** Yes, I know that Olivia on *Scandal* loves to lounge in these, but unless they're 100 percent cashmere and in a great color, it's like wearing your bathrobe out the door. Keep one or two that are luxe and lose the rest, especially the ones that are snagged or pilled. You're not foolin' anyone; we all know you're just trying to cover your butt and hips. Find a more stylish way to do it.

5. **Maternity clothes.** Are you pregnant? Are you planning to be tomorrow? If not, then why are still crawling into your Motherhood Maternity garb? Surely there is someone who can use your old pregnancy duds. Hand them down! Anything with "A Pea in the Pod" label—unless you have a bun in the oven—is off-limits.

6. **Mom jeans.** High-waisted, baggy, and universally unflattering. If they're stonewashed, that's reason enough to kick them to the curb. I never realized how butt-ugly they were until I got a pair of dark skinny jeans. Trust me, your derriere will thank you.

7. **Mid-calf skirts** (unless they are fitted, pencil skirts). Are you Amish? These skirts are not long, they're not short, they're somewhere ambiguously in the middle. They're confused. Shorten them or say goodbye.

8. **Boxy, clunky shoes.** I don't mean a cute platform or wedge; I mean a work boot, or anything that a nurse or a ninety-year-old might wear. Unless, of course, you prefer looking like a Pilgrim?

9. **Any vinyl or pleather handbags.** Basically, if it's shiny and likely to catch fire, you need to chuck it.

10. **Anything with an elastic waist**. Whether it's a dress, a skirt, a pair of pants, get rid of it. I understand that they s-t-r-e-t-c-h, but they also encourage your waist to get wider without you even noticing. The only elastic waists I have in my life now are on my silk pj's. Same goes for anything with a drawstring: ditch!

Learning to dress yourself

Recently, I've spent a lot of time with my toddler, trying to teach her how to put on her own shirt, pants, and shoes—all the basics of getting herself dressed in the morning, like a "big girl." That's when it dawned on me: I had no idea anymore how to dress myself. I could use a tutorial, too. An occasion or event would pop up (bat mitzvah, PTA meeting, cocktail party), and I'd run around my apartment in a panic. I had no clue what I should wear. My closet was a dark, scary place. What to do? Channel my inner bitch! I realized that every outfit I wore had to project power, confidence, and a touch of yeah-you-wish-you-were-me attitude. It's not as hard as you think.

The fifth-grade get-together. Why do PTAs insist on throwing these meet-and-greet dinners every back-to-school season? Mine are usually at night, in a restaurant/bar or someone's palatial apartment that's much neater, cleaner, and better decorated (is that a freakin' Picasso?) than mine. It's the first opportunity the other parents have to pass judgment on who you are, so you better be on your best bitch behavior. Consider a **dark-wash straight-leg jean.** You can dress it up or down, and it says, "I'm a modern mom." I might wear it with a **heel, a blazer/tee combo, and a great "It" bag** (see below).

Wedding/christening/bris/bar mitzvah. Anything requiring clergy to be present. You cannot go wrong with **a well-tailored suit** or a **simple sheath**. If it's a daytime affair, color is appropriate. Think **pretty pastels or neutrals**, nothing too bright or, God forbid, neon (this wasn't even a good option in the eighties). If it's an evening event that requires more dressy attire, I like **a little black dress** with a hint of sparkle over it, like a beaded jacket or wrap. Always carry a clutch and wear heels—these will help to pull your look together. You don't want to be toting a tote when you're asked to make a toast.

Cocktail or holiday party. Again, you can't go too far off track with **a black dress, pantsuit, or skirt** (knee-length or above-the-knee). Since it's an after-dark event, I say show a little skin: a **plunging V-neck sweater** or **an open-necked blouse**. You can also do sparkle and color, especially for the office Christmas bash. Just don't overdo the glitter or pile on too much jewelry. I'm a less is more kinda girl: one or two show-stopping pieces will do just fine. Choose the rhinestone earrings *or* the rhinestone necklace, not both. You want to look party-ready, not like a Christmas tree decorated by a six-year-old armed with twenty boxes of tinsel.

Date night with the hubby. Brian always notices if I make an effort, i.e., blow out my hair, put on makeup, and wear something that's figure-conscious. Flirty is the key word—an outfit that shows off your curves and cleavage, so he doesn't forget why he married you in the first place. I like a **soft, touchable sweater, a sexy, short skirt**, or for a more casual night out, **a silk sleeveless blouse/tank** and jeans. Think back to the way you dressed when you first started dating. Tap into that; break out the old photos if you need to refresh your memory. For God's sake, woman, sex yourself up!

Business meeting. Working from home most of the time, I used to just jump on a conference call in my sweats and slippers. Needless to say, I got a little out of practice with dressing to impress. When you're meeting clients, investors, or other professionals, you need to look like a grown-up again. Think **tailored, conservative clothing**, either **pants** or a **skirt** is fine, as long as the color and pattern aren't extreme. Of course, if you're in a creative field, you've got more options: an artist or a photographer can certainly go bolder. Basically, you want to be sure to call attention to your ideas and expertise—not what you're wearing.

Owning an "It" Bag

Not everyone can afford to spend a month's pay on a purse—God knows, I couldn't for years and years; and, if you ask my hubby, I still can't—we have three kids who outgrow their clothes hourly. I do, however, own a classic Chanel bag that belonged to my grandmother, so it's doubly fabulous: vintage and from my favorite lady in the world!

If you weren't fortunate enough to inherit one, then do peruse consignment shops, thrift stores, even tag sales. A friend of mine recently scored a Birkin at someone's backyard estate sale! Also, never underestimate places like T.J.Maxx or Century21—who knew they stocked Gucci, Balenciaga, Alexander McQueen, Stella McCartney, and Fendi at hundreds off the retail price? Cheap and chic—there's a reason these bags sell out and go for tons more on Ebay. Get 'em while you can. Same goes for sites like Rue La La and The RealReal. I'm also a huge fan of Target and H&M and their collaborations with designers like Phillip Lim, Zac Posen, Jimmy Choo, Balmain, Kenzo, and others.

If I'm in love with a bag, part of the fun for me is hunting it down on sale. My mother always taught me: nothing feels better than a bargain! But don't necessarily be swayed by the statusy label; it has to be a bag you will love and carry *almost* every day for years to come. I have a Celine tote that I never leave home without, and it was worth every penny.

A bitch needs a bag worthy of her confidence and charisma. In my case, it also has to be large so I can stow an extra pair of sneakers/flats, my daughter's favorite picture book, Ollie's acting script . . . you get the point. It's a "Bitch and Her Brood" carryall. But it's also very classy—and I do turn heads when I wear it. If it makes others green with envy, even better.

Five seconds to fabulous: instant ways to up your fashion quota when you're in a hurry

I have become the master of what I refer to as "instaglam," throwing on an accessory or two to jazz up an otherwise boring and basic outfit. I have a collection of things that add oomph—some are pricey, some are not, like the bright red pashmina wrap I bought off some guy on the street. Score! Here are a few things to have handy when you're on the run and need a quick fashion fix:

A great watch. Maybe one with a rose gold bracelet, a chic croc band, or a "diamond" face (crystals will do). Something that "arms" you with elegance and also ensures you're not late picking up your kid from daycare.

Jackie O sunglasses. Big round or square frames will make you look like a first lady—or at the very least a Hollywood star—as you navigate the aisles at the supermarket.

A chic wrap. Here's where you can add color to your LBD or a simple tee and jeans. I have a collection of wraps in assorted shades, everything from pastels and metallic gold to "proper" Burberry plain. You can't go wrong in wrapping up.

A statement necklace. These bold baubles can be anything from a single eye-popping pendant to strands of bright stones. Whenever I wear a boring navy sweater, I just put one on and feel like Cleopatra, even if I'm just headed to my son's baseball game.

Bangles. Whether you wear one funky, chunky one, or a stack of thin bangles in assorted metals or colors, these bracelets are bitch-worthy. I especially love when they jingle—so you other bitches know I'm coming!

A wide-brimmed sun hat. First of all, it keeps my dye job from going brassy. Secondly, it shades my face and keeps it from burning. Thirdly, it looks oh so glam in the spring or summer, like you've just come from the Kentucky Derby. Chic, chic, chic.

A silk scarf. I have a friend who tops every jacket, tee, and turtleneck with a colorful Hermès scarf; what she's spent on her collection could pay for a home in the Hamptons. But they don't need to be designer to be dramatic—I've seen great squares and oblongs at department stores for under $20. You can choose a single shade or go for intricate patterns. Whatever you choose, make sure it will add interest to your everyday look—think wearable art.

High heels and high chairs

I'm pretty sure I came out of the womb wearing stilettos. They have always been a ubiquitous part of my style. Nanadoll bought me my first pair for my bat mitzvah when I was thirteen. I thought I was the belle of the ball. If you told me that one day I'd trade in my signature shoe for a pair of UGGs, I would have called you delusional. Yet, there I was, seated in the auditorium for curriculum night, legs crossed, sporting footwear that belonged on an Eskimo, not a power mom. I tried to rationalize. Yes, they were comfy. Yes, they were warm. And, yes, it's certainly easier to race around in them. But me, of all people?

When I got home, I dug through my closet and found my favorite pair of Louboutins. I slipped them on. They pinched a little more than before I was pregnant, but I loved how they made me feel: fierce.

Over the years, I've come to realize that there are two types of women: those who "heel" and those who don't. My loafer-loving gal pals will tell me I'm crazy. They say that high heels maim and mangle your feet. Who needs that pain and suffering, isn't motherhood enough? But I think of it more as a mental exercise. When you wear heels, you walk taller, literally and figuratively. It's kind of hard for me to be a bitch wearing a ballet flat.

So, if it means I must suffer, then so be it! Billy Crystal's *Saturday Night Live* character Fernando knew what he was talking about when he said: "It is better to look good than to feel good."

I think every bitch needs a pair of heels in her life. They don't have to be sky-high—you don't want to look like you're walking on eggshells or be clinging to the walls for support. Keep it sane: a moderate two to three inches is fine. And bear in mind the following tips for staying on your toes:

- **You may need to go up a size or more,** especially if the shoe is pointy. Don't look at the number, just try them on and make sure your toes aren't bunched up.

- **Try on heels at the end of the day** when your feet tend to be more swollen—you'll get a more accurate read on how comfy (or not) they are.

- **Thicker soles equal more comfort,** which is why a lot of women love platform heels. They take some of the pressure off when you're walking.

- **Take a break.** Don't think you can survive a nine-to-five workday without taking your heels off. That's what the space under your desk is for!

- **Stretch your feet.** As soon as you get those shoes off, work out the kinks in your feet and ankles by pointing, flexing, and circling your feet. I also like to rub my feet (or have my hubby do it) at the end of a long day with a little peppermint-scented lotion.

- **Drugstore shoe inserts really *do* work.** The oval-shaped gel pads go under the ball of the foot, alleviating some of the pressure and preventing your feet from sliding forward and pinching. I'm also a fan of those little friction and blister cushions and always throw a few in my purse.

- **Learn to walk in them.** Yes, there is a science to it. Imagine there is a string attached to the top of your head and it's pulling you up as you walk—work that inner core and engage your calf muscles. This will keep your posture in line, your butt up and out, and your stride smooth. Lead with the ball of the foot, never with the heel or toes—this is what separates the pros from the amateurs. Take smaller steps and don't rush it. Remember, practice makes perfect: take your heels out for a test drive at home before you wear them out on the street.

- **Avoid slips and spills.** Supermodel Tyra Banks swears by this trick she learned during her Paris runway days: take a scissor (keep the blades closed) and score the bottom of your shoes, creating grooves. This will take off the slick gloss that's on the soles. And, frankly, Ty is one tough chick, so I'll believe whatever she says.

What to wear under there

Tempting as it was to stay in my roomy, soft nursing bras, they were doing nothing to boost my morale—or my boobs, for that matter. I came to realize that bitches need to rock their undergarments like a Victoria's Secret runway model:

- **Hide the granny panties.** I mean it; bury them in the back of your drawer. Think cut, color, and fabric: a thong, a bikini, or a high-cut hipster in lace, silk, or satin and in a wide-range of shades, from black and nude (it just sounds dirty!) to red-hot red.

- **Spanx are a mom's best friend.** I don't recommend you sharing that with your hubby (he doesn't need to see you parade around in your "shapewear"), but they have the uncanny ability to pack it in and flatten it out, thereby reducing your waist to the size of Scarlett O'Hara's. God bless a good girdle.

- I don't care if no one else sees it, **your bra should be sexy**. You know it's under there, even if no one else does. In my opinion, lace and satin are always good choices—I'd lay off the latex rubber unless kinky is your thing (more power to you!). Consider a wardrobe of at least seven different styles—one for each day of the week. Include a strapless, a sports bra, a padded push-up, a bralette (great for sleeping), a convertible, a demi, and a few of the va-va-va-voom variety.

Sizing up your bra size

After giving birth to Blake, my boobs ballooned. I truly have no idea what size they are anymore. Sometimes I look down at my chest and it's like a stranger's rack is staring back at me. "As moms, we all know what happens to your body after childbirth and as we age," says style expert Jene Luciani. "Gravity sends 'the girls' down toward our feet." And who knew that our bra size is constantly fluctuating: even the loss or gain of as little as five to ten pounds can change it. Jene recommends an annual bra fitting. "Make it a fun Mom's Day Out," she says. "Grab some girlfriends, some champagne, and a limo if your budget allows, pick your favorite specialty shop, and make a day of it. You'll all emerge a little perkier, I promise!"

Quite honestly, I had no idea how the whole bra size thing worked. What letter of the alphabet was I, C, D, DD? I had one of each in my drawer postpregnancy. So Jene enlightened me. Your bra size contains two important figures:

- An even number that represents the size of your rib cage (all the way around your back) and corresponds to the band size
- A letter that correlates to your cup size in relation to your band size

These two figures are in proportion to each other. While it sounds simple, it isn't. The band size doesn't necessarily equal the width of your rib cage. Often you take the rib cage measurement and will have to add one or two inches to get your actual band size. Also, your band size may vary depending on the manufacturer and styles. A 34 in one style may feel just right, while a 34 in another may be too tight. Your band size is estimated *based* on the diameter of your rib cage, but it isn't an exact science.

What's also inconsistent is your band size *in relation to* your cup size. For example, an A cup on a 32 band size is not the same as an A cup on the 34 band size, and so on. Instead, the size of, or volume held by, an A cup changes depending on the band size. What this means practically is that if you go down a band size, you can generally go up in cup size, and vice versa, and achieve a similar fit, because each of these combinations of "sizes" is made to hold the same volume of breast tissue.

DIY: Calculating Your Bra Size

Step 1: First, wrap the tape measure (the sewing kind, not the toolbox kind) around your rib cage, just below your bust (be sure to exhale first) and take the measurement. Since bra band sizes are even numbers, round up to the nearest even number. For example, if you measure at an odd 31 inches, round up to 32.

Step 2: Next, wrap the tape measure around the fullest part of your bust. Then subtract your band size from this number and use the difference in inches to calculate your cup size. For example, if your bust measurement is one inch larger than your band size, your cup size will most likely be an A; if your bust measurement is two inches larger than your band size, your cup size will most likely be a B; and so on.

Note that sizes vary widely by brand, so this is only meant to be a guideline. *Always* try bras on at the store and move around in them. The band shouldn't be too snug, but you want to be sure it's not too loose, as the band (not the straps) will provide your girls with the support they need. Lift your arms to see if the band stays in place. It's okay if the band moves slightly, but it should not move so much that it lands between your shoulder blades. If the band feels comfortable, slip the straps down off your shoulders to check that it is providing the proper support.

To ensure you have the correct cup size, look for bulges or loose fabric. Bend over to ensure the girls stay snug inside the cups, so you can avoid the potential for future wardrobe malfunctions.

Bitch of the Day:

"I can't afford a whole new wardrobe."

Honey, unless you're a millionaire (or married to one), I wouldn't expect you to go out and replace every single thing in your closet. Start with one or two new pieces that a) can go from day to night, so you'll get a lot of mileage out of them; and b) flatter you and make you feel good about yourself. You can build on that. And the next time someone asks you what you want for your b-day, anniversary, Christmas, Ground Hog's Day, etc., say a gift card to your fave store. As Nanadoll would say, "Use it in good health!"

STEP 5
EXTREME MAKEOVER, BITCHY MAMA STYLE

"I'm totally not against plastic surgery. Trust me, honey, if I take this bra off, you will tell me I need to get them done."

—*Kim Kardashian*

My kids remind me all the time that I will be old when my hair goes gray. Little do they know I went gray at thirty (my father went gray early, and I have many of his traits, including his blue eyes, height, and terrible handwriting). So, yes, I color my hair every four weeks and I get Botox twice a year. You would not believe how long it takes to get that appointment at the plastic surgeon's office, which means I'm not the only one! Trust me, your fresh-faced friends are lying if they tell you they don't "clean up" every now and then. It takes a village—or at the very least a team of trusted professionals—to look awake and not feel ancient. If I didn't treat myself to the occasional tune-up, I'd have luggage—not just bags—under my eyes.

Before I became "ambitchous," I walked around with roots, unpolished nails bitten to the quick, and feet that felt like sandpaper. I'd keep telling myself I'd get to it, but I never did. I just couldn't justify it. I had three kids; I had work; I had dinner to make and endless errands to run. If my nail polish was chipped, did it really matter? The answer is yes, it matters. It matters because this is the image you're projecting to the world: I'm a mess because I'm a mom. It matters because it shows how low you put yourself on your list of priorities. It matters because it affects your self-esteem.

So, I made myself an appointment with a hairstylist. Step one: cover the grays. Step two: get a decent cut (anything but the mom lob). Step three: schedule a weekly blowout for maintenance. That blowout is a must (my hairdresser is also my therapist). I'll also do a gel mani/pedi every other week, an occasional massage and facial, and a weed-whacking wax on my legs, bikini line, and brows. No woman (unless she's sixteen) wakes up naturally gorgeous. You owe this to yourself. It's great to be comfortable in your own skin, just make sure that skin is unblemished, devoid of wrinkles, and as soft as a baby's bottom.

Five-minute makeup (that doesn't look it)

I've dubbed my morning routine "Hurricane Lyss"—see it in action, and you'd declare a national emergency. There's no easy way to drag three kids out of bed and get them dressed, fed, and out the door by 8:00 a.m. If Ollie gets to school wearing two sneakers that match, it's a good day. I used to run out sans makeup with my hair in a matted mess. Now, I've gotten a grip on it. I set my alarm an hour early to "wake before the quake" (my friend June Ambrose coined the term) and spend that time dedicated to myself. But, even when I only have five minutes to spare, this makeup magic from beauty expert Laura Geller is lightning quick and looks great:

1 minute: Apply foundation to cover skin flaws on the go—by using a large brush, you will cover more area faster.

30 seconds: Use a large brush to apply a thin layer of translucent powder to set and "matte-ify."

30 seconds: Using a blush brush, sweep a rosy blusher on the apples of your cheeks.

30 seconds: Use a waterproof liner along the upper lash line only. This will open the eyes up and make you look more awake.

30 seconds: Swipe on a natural, dark mascara—nothing too thick that will clump and harden throughout the day. Look for one that volumizes and lengthens but feels light on the eye.

1 minute: Brush brows into shape. Use a brow gel pencil to fill in any areas that are sparse. Use a spoolie brush to soften the line.

1 minute: Apply lipstick in a shade close to your natural lip color; it will look like you, only better. To keep color from kissing off, top with a coat of gloss.

Hair in a hurry

Dig in the bottom of my purse and you'll find a collection of elastics, hair ties, butterfly clips, and that dreaded eighties staple, the hair scrunchie. I have a collection of them that are older than my teenage son. In my prebitch period, a scrunchie was about all I could muster for my mane. I'd either pull my hair back into a pony or pile it high on my head in a matted mess (definitely not the inspiration behind the messy bun look). There was no "style" to my 'do—just desperation. My mother was appalled: my long, thick hair was her pride and joy, and her bragging rights. "Elyssa," she kvetched, "what happened to you?"

Life happened to me; motherhood happened to me. But Nanadoll was right, as much as it pains me to admit it: my hair had always been my crowning glory. I needed a style that would work on days when I had no time to spare. I turned to Edward Tricomi, master stylist and cofounder of Warren-Tricomi Salons, to teach me a few tricks.

The modern messy bun. Use a brush or your fingers to smooth your hair and bring it to the top of your head—think troll hair. Now, twist the hair until it forms a loose bun on the top of your head. It's okay if your hair is a little dirty or a few strays slip free— this look is supposed to be loose. Use a clip, a few bobby pins, or a hair elastic to secure the bun in place. I like to leave a few fringy ends out, creating a fan effect. If you want to get real fancy, borrow one of your daughter's sparkly hair clips to dress it up (rhinestones, yes; bows, no). Done and done!

The grown-up pony. If you got to shower this a.m., lucky you! You can start with clean hair. If not, no worries. This look masks all. Brush your hair back into a smooth ponytail; a spritz of Warren-Tricomi Flexible Hair Spray will sleek and tame any frizzies. I like to wear my pony high, at the crown of the head, but you can wear yours anywhere that works for you, from the nape to midhead. Secure with an elastic. Take a small section of the tail (about an inch wide) and wrap it around the elastic several times, until you reach the ends. Tuck under or use a bobby pin to secure. You can also braid this section and wrap the braid around—your call. It just makes your pony look more polished.

The braid–bun mashup. First, comb through any tangles. Separate the hair into three sections. Braid very loosely, allowing strands to slip free or pop out. Now, secure two of the three sections at the end of the braid with an elastic band, leaving the last one free. Pull the loose strand at the end of the braid, pushing up the rest of the hair until you've formed a bun. Tuck the loose strand under, then place a large bobby pin horizontally to secure the bun in place. If you want this to look neater, you can add more pins—I prefer that messy-hair-I-don't-care feel. Spray with finishing spray to hold.

The "hair-band." Using a teasing brush, part hair naturally. Section out two face-framing sections of hair, ½ inch to 1 inch in thickness. Pull the rest of your hair back into a ponytail. Now, with an elastic band, secure the two sections at the nape of your neck. Release the pony so your hair now falls loosely over the hair-band. Mist lightly with a finishing spray to add shine and hold.

Quick root cover-up

In my humble opinion, those pesky little gray hairs that pop up are the root of all evil. Hair grows at a rate of about ½ inch a month, which means you have four weeks before your roots begin to show. I try to hit the hair salon before they surface, but some mornings I wake up and there they are, staring me in the face. It's like they grew in overnight just to piss me off. When I don't have time to get a professional touch-up, these tricks will tide me over until I can get an appointment with my stylist.

- **Switch your part.** Simply combing your hair in a different direction or with a zigzag part can hide grays for a few days.

- **Pick up a root cover-up product** in the drugstore (like Clairol Nice 'N Easy Root Touchup or L'Oréal Paris Root Rescue). Most will last about three to four weeks, so you can find the time to make that salon appointment. You paint, brush, or spray the product on problem areas and get instant camouflage.

- If your issue is dark roots in blond hair, **add highlights** from a kit to break up the line and make growout less noticeable.

- **Try a root touch-up powder kit** (like Color Wow, Root Touch Up from Madison Reed, or John Frieda Root Blur). They look like large eye shadows with a stiff brush, and the powder adheres without feeling sticky. Another plus: you can also use it on thinning areas.

- Edward Tricomi also suggests **using mascara in a pinch**—just swipe it on over those gray strands, and no one will be the wiser.

Bitch of the Day

"I think I'm going bald! I just had my baby, and my hair is falling out in clumps!"

Been there, done that. My drain looked like one of those little furry pom-poms everyone is using to accessorize their bags. There's a very good explanation for it: after you give birth, your estrogen levels take a nosedive, and a lot more hair follicles enter the resting stage—meaning your head keeps shedding while nothing is growing. So, don't be surprised if you see clumps coming out in the shower or in your brush. In about six months to a year, your hair should be back to its normal thickness. In the meantime, I'd experiment with some new cuts and highlights to add volume and dimension. This too shall pass, I promise—might as well get a cute new 'do out of it.

STEP 6
YOU'VE GOT A MOUTH . . . USE IT

"These days, I strive to be a bitch, because not being one sucks. Not being a bitch means not having your voice heard."

—Margaret Cho

So, I'm in line with my daughter at the supermarket checkout, and this mom with her perfect hair and her perfect baby in her ridiculously expensive Euro stroller is giving me a dirty look. I'm not really sure why: maybe it had to do with the fact that Blakey was pitching an I-need-my-afternoon-nap hissy fit, and her tantrum was clearly disturbing Perfect Mom's delicate ears.

I stared the woman down, then I spoke up. "Yes, my child self-destructs every day around 3:00 p.m. when she's cranky, tired, hungry, and generally in a foul mood. Are you telling me yours doesn't ever have a meltdown?"

She ignored me, so I knew exactly what I had to do: sing. I started crooning at the top of my lungs, "If you're happy and you know it, clap your hands!" Blake stopped crying. Her face broke into a huge smile, and she was suddenly giddy with laughter. We were now singing and clapping together, having a grand old time. And all that noise woke up perfect baby . . . who began to wail hysterically. Now look who has to deal with a crying kid. It's fun, isn't it? I walked out of Whole Foods triumphant—take that!

The world is filled with judgy moms, nasty naysayers, and relentless naggers—that's just a fact. You have to adapt a bitch mentality when dealing with them; I'm Teflon, honey: your snide remarks and evil glances just slide right off me. You can't touch this! Don't be afraid to say something back—sometimes grown-ups and not just children need a scolding. I'm not one to keep silent when someone is attacking me or my child for being who we are. It's the bitch in me at its best. There are nice ways to do it, polite ways, and even creative ones to get your point across—like breaking into song in the supermarket. Just don't stand there letting someone pass judgment on you or throw shade. Life is too short for haters to have the winning hand.

Of course, some negativity comes from unexpected places, like your own family. A friend of mine called me complaining, "My sister-in-law thinks I spoil my kids. She says I'm a terrible mom!" I told her to take deep breath. "You're a great mom," I reminded her. "And just because you bought your kid every Shopkins on the shelf for her birthday doesn't mean you're evil. Indulgent maybe, but not evil."

Here's how I handle situations like the above: my kid, my rules. And I mean that: no one gets to tell me how to parent. I don't care if you're my husband's blood relative; that doesn't give you the right to interfere. If I want your opinion, I will ask for it, period. Until that day, can we please agree to disagree and I don't have to hear about it?

Another close friend has an eight-year-old son who was horribly homesick while he was at sleepaway camp. She picked him up two weeks early, only to be met with a tirade from her mother-in-law. "You have scarred him for life!" she insisted. "He will forever feel like a sissy because you allowed him to chicken out and go home."

I shook my head in disbelief: is sleepaway camp prison? Do our kids have to serve a sentence of eight weeks if they are miserable and miss their mommy? I know a lot of moms who preach tough love, especially when it comes to sleepaway camp, but no one knows your kid better than you. You get to call the shots, not anyone else. You're entitled to your opinions, but I don't have to agree with them. And I certainly don't deserve to have them shoved down my throat.

My friend cowered; she let her mother-in-law get the last word. She felt guilty and terrible, which is exactly what her mother-in-law hoped she would feel. I wanted to shake her and yell, "Snap out of it!" This is not how a bitch handles a cutting comment. She faces it head-on.

My own family is much more subtle. I just get the snarky backhanded compliments, like, "Lyss, is that a new dress? Is that in style these days?" There's just that little hint of disapproval that can grate on my nerves. Fellow moms do it to me, too. I'm picking Jax up from baseball practice and I get, "Lyss, you look so tired. Is everything okay?" I know you're not really concerned about my health and well-being, you just want me to know you think I look like shit. I get it.

When faced with friction, you have two options: ignore or engage. Both are effective; both require a backbone. It depends a lot on who you're dealing with. Sometimes I just fantasize what I might say, and I feel a lot better.

The meddling mom/mom-in-law says: "I would never let my kids eat candy for breakfast! That's horrible parenting."

The inner bitch thinks: "Well, little Johnny was trying to eat the dog's food yesterday, so I see this as a vast improvement. Thanks for the words of wisdom, Granny!" (The age dig is a nice touch.)

The calm, cool bitch responds: "Well, Johnny prefers Kit Kats, but we switched to Snickers Dark, because dark chocolate is a source of procyanidins, which function as antioxidants in the body, and there's protein from the peanuts. And it's important to include protein in the diet, as you know."

The psycho sister/sis-in-law says: "I tried on my high school jeans and they still fit. Don't you wish you were as tiny as me?"

The inner bitch thinks: "Sure do! And you will, too, after you've had three kids and your ass is too big to fit through the door, much less into your old jeans. But cling to what you have—it'll be gone soon enough."

The calm, cool bitch responds: "Ah, high school, I remember it well! Aren't those the 'mom' jeans that went out of style fifteen years ago?"

The snarky soccer mom says: "Aw, it's too bad little Lisa missed that goal. Have you had her eyes checked?"

The inner bitch thinks: "You're so kind to be concerned. I know you have your hands full with your own kid's lack of coordination. I hear occupational therapy works wonders."

The calm, cool bitch responds: "Research tells us that losing games is good for children and helps them develop into empathetic, well-adjusted people—something we should all strive to be."

The know-it-all teacher says: "Your son failed his math quiz—clearly you're not helping him learn his multiplication tables at home."

The inner bitch thinks: "Of course! What do I know? I only have a master's degree from Yale and a doctorate from Princeton. Can I see your credentials?"

The calm, cool bitch responds: "I appreciate your concern, and we can work on this together. We will spend more time with him at home going over it, and perhaps you can find some time in your busy schedule to work with him as well."

Your nagging neighbor says: "Your hydrangea bushes are quite an eyesore! I guess gardening isn't your forte?"

The inner bitch thinks: "Actually, it's not. But you know what is? Suing people for slander."

The calm, cool bitch responds: "You're right. Maybe you could give me some pointers—since you love digging up dirt."

Your unthinking hubby says: "What did you do all day?"

The inner bitch thinks: "Oh, not much. Just sat around in my pj's, ate bonbons, and binge-watched *Odd Mom Out*. Isn't it amazing how dinner gets made by itself and your children arrive home from school and sports practice on their own? It's magic!"

The calm, cool bitch responds: "Let's see, I did housework, volunteered at the school library, drove the kids to Little League, and whipped up a gourmet dinner. Yup, that about sums it up. Can you top that?"

A Case for Keeping Your Cool

Most of the time, when people are negative, it's because of them, not you. They are insecure, afraid, angry, depressed, and frustrated, and they choose to target you in an attempt to make themselves feel bigger and better. I try and practice the 10-second rule: I give myself that tiny amount of time to take a deep breath, count to ten, and think before I react. I might *want* to say one of the above zingers, but it might be more effective to simply walk away. No reaction can be the best course of action; it's like dousing a flame with water.

Consider who is doing the dissing. Is it a close friend, a relative, a coworker, a spouse? All the more reason to tread lightly and remove yourself from the situation. A recent study by researchers at Baruch College found that the silent treatment is truly the best way to handle rude and offensive individuals. Why? Because it's their goal to push your buttons. If that's the case, don't give them what they want. Be ice, ice baby.

Say what you mean, mean what you say

I believe you can't just talk the talk; you also have to back it up with action. I have a friend who tells me, "I'm so sick of my PTA copresident dumping thankless tasks on me! I'm gonna tell her I'm done!" Does she? Let's put it this way: she canceled on lunch with me last week because she was stuffing 700 invites for the annual auction into envelopes. She does a lot of complaining, but the words are empty if she doesn't act on them.

Being honest and upfront with everyone in your life is Bitch101. You can do it with tact, diplomacy, and delicacy, but by all means express yourself in a way that conveys your true feelings. I do this with my friends, my employees, my hubby, and my kids. There is never a time I regret it, because it comes from a place of integrity. People will respect you more for it. A lot of women will simply restate the obvious or go with the consensus. That's fine if you're trying to win a popularity contest. I'm not. I'm trying to live my life as genuinely as I can and get through each day with my sanity intact. Bullshit has no place in my life, nor should it in yours. Just sayin'.

Bitch of the Day

*"I cannot deal with my nanny! She uses the cell phone
I gave her to make calls 'back home' and hands me a
grocery list every week of foods she wants me to stock in the
fridge for her. I know my one-year-old adores her, but am I
supposed to just let her get away with murder?"*

No, you're not. You need to sit this chick down and tell
her who's the boss in no uncertain terms. If she doesn't
like it, too bad—there's several hundred nannies out there
who are eager to take her place. Ask your friends; they'll
be happy to put the word out and find you a new one. And
your baby will be fine with a new, caring nanny. You are a
victim of babysitter abuse, and it's time to put an end to
it. I'm tough as nails on this issue; diva nannies need not
apply at my place. Give her a warning, then if she doesn't
shape up, ship her out. I promise you will find a loving,
caring new nanny who doesn't walk all over you.

STEP 7
SURROUND YOURSELF WITH BITCHES

"We've got to remember to have a glass of wine and escape for a little TLC of our own without the guilt. Lesson learned."

—*Rebecca Minkoff, fashion designer*

There's power in numbers, so you want to gather your troops around you. Bitches love company. We count on it to keep us on track. I don't know what I would do without my girlfriends (but it might involve a very high bridge). Over the years, friends have come into and out of my life. The ones that remain share my philosophy and have my back. The others . . . well, they've either turned out to be frenemies (see below) or proved themselves unworthy of me.

I have friends I'll text every day and others I won't see for weeks or months at a time. But they're there when I need them, bitchy, beautiful, and bound by one common goal: to be the very best moms and human beings we all can be. I can call, and no matter how much time has passed, we pick up exactly where we left off. A true friend doesn't keep tabs on who called whom or who bought lunch last. They simply relish the time with you, because we make each other sane and whole.

As I get older (and older), I realize the value of a power posse. A Yale study found that the people in the over-sixty set are 45 percent more likely to die if they feel alone or isolated. Friends are good for your health! I don't know about you, but that's enough reason to organize a Girls' Night Out once a week. I like to think of my girlfriends as a sisterhood, a tribe. Meredith Grey had Cristina Yang; Laverne had Shirley. I have a long list of women that I can turn to for comfort and support or just plain laughs. I think we all need a handful of friends, each with a different role in our lives:

The Tell-It-To-You-Straight Friend. She will not mince words; if you have spinach stuck in your teeth, she'll tell you. If you chose the wrong wallpaper for your kitchen, she'll say so—lovingly, of course. You can ask her anything, and she will take a moment, think it through, then respond with exactly what you need to make your own, smart, educated choices. She's your sounding board and your moral compass, and you can trust that her advice is sincere.

The Goof-Off Girlfriend. Need a day of doing absolutely nothing to de-stress? She's your gal. She's happy to just hang at home, watch Netflix, order in pizza. When you want to decompress, simply DM or text her and she'll arrive, bearing boxes of cupcakes and bottles of rosé for the ultimate lazy afternoon. When you're down, she knows exactly how to lift you up: *I Love Lucy* reruns!

The Bitch Playlist

When you need to dance it out, drown out the sound of your kids trying to kill each other, or tell everyone on the planet to PISS OFF, just pump up one of these jams. I promise, you'll feel much better.

"Respect" by Aretha Franklin
"Q.U.E.E.N." by Janelle Monáe featuring Erykah Badu
"A Woman's Worth" by Alicia Keys
"I'm Every Woman" by Chaka Khan
"Run the World (Girls)" by Beyoncé
"No More Drama" by Mary J. Blige
"Doo Wop That Thing" by Lauryn Hill
"Fly" by Nicki Minaj featuring Rihanna
"Love Myself" by Hailey Steinfeld
"Fuck You" by Lily Allen (I'm seriously considering making this my ringtone!)

The Noted Authority Friend. She has all the answers: what to do when your kid is running a fever; how to make anything from scratch; what you can (and can't) claim on your tax deductions. This summa cum laude sister will do all the homework and research for you—that is, if she doesn't know the answer already. She's your first call when faced with a conundrum—and for good reason.

The Sexpert Friend. Think Samantha on *Sex and the City*. This woman has been around the block more than once and is happy to give you some tips and tricks. Usually divorced or single, she's a fountain of info and is happy to let you live vicariously through her exploits, especially when it's been weeks since you and the hubby hit the hay (a newborn will do that to ya!). Who needs to read *50 Shades* when she's on your speed dial?

The Emergency Friend. Who would you call if you were arrested? You guessed it—this gal pal is calm and cool in any crisis. She knows how to talk you off a ledge, and what to do when the shit hits the fan and you're out of options. In-laws popping in for a surprise visit? She'll help you hide all the mess under the couch so no one is the wiser. Forgot about the bake sale at school? She'll bring you a pie without batting an eye. What would you do without her?

The Party Girl Friend. She's someone you can count on to be your plus-one whenever you need one, even if it's last minute. She's always up for a good time and will gladly sample any new restaurant, bar, or lounge you've been dying to try. She's the one person who reminds you that you weren't always changing diapers, and she knows how to get your ass off the couch and out the door—with the promise of fun, fun, fun.

Girls' Night In

Every so often, I desperately need to kick back with my closest pals for an at-home bitching session. Case in point: a week prior to my son's bar mitzvah. I was stressed to the breaking point. So, I shooed the hubby and kids out of the house and called in the troops. You don't need a detailed game plan (frankly, a couple bottles of wine and some cheese and crackers will do ya), but I'm a details person. I love to throw a memorable ladies-only party. And don't we all deserve it? Here are some tips to make your next girls' night in a memorable one:

Set the mood. I like candles—they not only create a relaxing atmosphere, but they also cover up the stench of two boys, a diaper pail, and a dog. I might also fill some vases with fresh flowers, break out pretty table linens, and use the good crystal stemware instead of paper cups.

Provide the entertainment. Rent a few great chick flicks (*Bridget Jones's Baby* for laughs; *Magic Mike* if you're feeling raunchy) and veg out in front of the TV with your friends. When's the last time any of you got to command the remote?

Arrange for at-home pampering. A masseuse or a manicurist that makes house calls is always a hit. A friend of mine even arranged for a yoga instructor to lead a class in her living room. Personally, I think a hairstylist that does blowouts for all would be lovely.

Serve eats that are treats. These do not include Girl Scout cookies, Jell-O shots, or anything that comes in a box labeled "Kraft." I'm talking good cheese, good wine, decadent chocolate. My friend brought a huge box of champagne-flavored gummy bears to my last soiree to share. Alcohol + sugar—how can you go wrong?

Let the good times flow. Make sure you have a good assortment of wine, some prosecco, and a fully stocked bar. You can even whip up a pitcher of sangria or create a signature cocktail for the evening (see Bitchitini recipe on page 79).

Hand out goodie bags. I believe that every party hostess should leave her guests with a souvenir of the evening. I'd stock mine with a mini bottle of champagne, some French macarons, a pretty nail polish or lip gloss, and, of course, a copy of a great book. (I highly recommend the book in your hands!)

Bitch Recipe Box Bonus

The Bitchitini

One day I was in the kitchen with my girlfriend, cutting up watermelon (and picking out the pits) for our kids' snack and chugging down glasses of watermelon juice. "Ya know," I commented, "this would taste even better with a shot of vodka or a splash of rosé." We got out the ingredients, and the Bitchitini was born! It's now become the cocktail of choice when I have friends over—or when I've had a tough day and need to unwind.

Ingredients:
3 ounces rosé wine
1 ounce watermelon vodka, such as Smirnoff Watermelon
1 ounce fresh watermelon juice

Directions:
Shake watermelon vodka, watermelon juice, and rosé wine in a cocktail shaker with ice.
Pour into a chilled cocktail glass.
Garnish with a watermelon chunk.

Bitch of the Day

"I do not have a minute to myself; my three-year-old literally follows me into the toilet when I go pee."

At least he lets you pee. My three-year-old will fling herself in front of the bathroom door and refuse to let me in if it means interrupting her mommy and me time. You are entitled to a potty break and so much more. Not even a Supermom can be expected to be on call 24/7, 365 days a year. You have to make the time for yourself or you'll be no good to anyone. Stop complaining about it and do it.

As Natalie Klein, co-owner of Hot Moms Club, says, "It is a twenty-four-hour job, whether you work at home or work in an office. It's a job with no financial gain and no days off. You are often underappreciated, misunderstood, and you can't just quit. Take care of yourself; whether you need a night of trashy TV, or Xanax, or tequila, or ice cream and cookies. Have your hot massage therapist on speed dial. Whatever it takes for you to recharge, because it's the most important and most rewarding job of your life."

STEP 8
TRAIN YOUR KIDS

*"Motherhood is nonstop madness, emotionally
unpredictable in ways you've never imagined. It is often
thankless and faceless, and if you're doing your job right,
your kids shouldn't even notice 99% of the time that they
have an excellent parent. They push as hard as they
can, and it's our job to push back, because the world
does not suffer fools easily and the consequences in real
life are enormous compared to any limits, controls, or
punishments we can set as parents."*

—Veronica Webb

Training your kids is essential—and I don't just mean on the potty. Getting them out of diapers was a lot easier than teaching my trio to give me five minutes of uninterrupted time on the phone. You need to educate them to the fact that mommy has a life and is a human being, not a machine. I am capable of emotions, exhaustion, and the occasional shit fit. I break and I cry, and I require sleep, food, and a shower once in a while to keep going. Without these essentials, I'm no good to anybody— not my family, not myself.

Every single day I am juggling 101 balls at once trying not to let one drop. I am running on Dunkin' and swigging Starbucks by the gallon; caffeine is my drug of choice. And yet, my three simply don't get it. I am not their underling, their emotional punching bag, or their handmaiden. The old me would have shrugged it off: kids will be kids, ya gotta love 'em (do you have a choice?). The new me put my children in a bitch-inspired boot camp: you will appreciate what I do, you will respect me, and you will pitch in. Why? Because I said so. And as any bitch will tell you, that's reason enough.

Being a little tough as a parent will not kill them. Kids are not that fragile; they can take the disappointment of no sweets before supper, schlepping their own backpacks on the walk to school, and putting their dishes in the sink. Saying no to them won't scar them for life, nor will refusing to buy your teenager the new iPhone the minute it comes out. Whining, complaining, crying will get you nowhere—I've heard it all, and I'm immune to the kvetching. My Ollie always wants to negotiate—he's king of the counteroffer—and is either going to direct movies or be a ballbusting litigator. He tries to bargain with me: "Mom, I will do my homework *after* you let me stay up and watch *Saturday Night Live*." Homework at 1:00 a.m., really?

Each of my children has their own big, bold personality. Jax wants to play for MLB and can't understand why school needs to interfere with practice. But Blakey, my baby, is the most independent one of all. I'm convinced she's the reincarnation of my grandmother, a beauty with a personality like no other who knows what she wants and won't take no for an answer. I adore each and every one of them for who they are, even if they do have a knack for pushing my buttons. I try to be a cool mom and not nag incessantly, but sometimes there's no way around it. I'm not asking for that much, simply to be treated as I treat them: with love, devotion, and sympathy whenever they ask for it. You got a boo-boo? Mommy will kiss it better. If Mommy's got a boo-boo (i.e., a splitting migraine), can we please keep the noise down to a dull roar?

Beyond that, it's simply a matter of communication: this is how it's gonna go because Mom rules the roost. I suggest creating 10 Commandments for Kids and displaying them prominently on the fridge. When you're eighteen and no longer living under my roof, we'll talk. But for now:

1. **Do your best every day in every way.** That means being honest, good, and caring people.

2. **Be respectful to your parents**—no mouthing off or declaring how annoying we are. We gave you life; you owe us big-time.

3. **Be a kind and gentle sibling:** don't beat up your sister/brother. I don't care if she/he started it. Blood is thicker than Hershey's syrup.

4. **Be polite**—no belching, farting, or picking your nose in public, unless you *really* can't help it. Say please, thank you, and excuse me. They're not dirty words.

5. **Do your homework** by the time it's due (not a few days later). Even if you have to miss the season finale of *America's Got Talent* (that's what TiVo is for).

6. **Be a team player and a good sport** . . . and carry your own equipment. I'm Wonder Woman, not "bat girl."

7. **Clean up after yourselves**—mom is not your maid, and you can all make your beds after you sleep in them. Dirty laundry goes in the laundry bag, and your plates go in the sink. Your brother's head does not go in the toilet.

8. **Lend a hand.** That means when your mother is freaking out and on the edge of a breakdown, ask what you can do to help her. Do your chores without breaking into the chain gang song from *Les Mis*. (Ollie, you know who I'm talking to.)

9. **Be responsible.** If I say, "Text me when you get to Billy's house," I mean it. If I tell you to hold your little sister's hand on the beach, don't leave her at the edge of the ocean to go boogie boarding. Put the seat down after you pee so I don't fall in. Is that too much to ask?

10. **Be you.** Never lose sight of who you are and what makes you unique and special. I gave birth to three incredible kids who will grow up to be three incredible adults. I may yell, threaten, and nag, but I love you with all my heart and soul.

Set your boundaries

Just like children, moms need time-outs every day. A happy mom equals a happy family. My kids need to understand that I have a life outside of them; *most* of my world may revolve around their every whim and whine, but a tiny percentage has to be for me, me, me. For some reason, this never goes over well. Someone either clings to my ankle as I'm trying to get out the door (usually not the little one) or texts me every 10 seconds once I've left. I'm entitled to meet a friend for coffee, a client for lunch, and their father for a date night. If this interferes with their plans, I'm sorry, but it's nonnegotiable. Grandma, dad, or a sitter can be on call for two hours. I promise, you will not *die* if someone other than the woman who bore you has to tuck you into bed.

Kids will naturally push back when you make them do something they don't want to do (which is just about anything I ask). You're trying to rein them in, and they want to be independent. I get it, and independence is a good thing, but not when your toddler is determined to style her own hair and you're late to a pediatrician appointment. I tell fellow moms they need to be realistic: your child is not perfect. They are going to screw up, be fresh, freak out. On a recent trip to grandma's house, the back seat erupted into World War III: crying, yelling, and kicking. Unless you have nerves of steel or noise-canceling headphones, you're going to have to grit your teeth and listen to their griping. You know you want to scream about the traffic, too. At least someone should be allowed to vent.

However, that doesn't mean you have to stand for any disrespect. I want my kids to have fun with me. We frequently have our own date days/nights when we go to a show, a movie, or a cool new ice cream place in the city. But I make something perfectly clear to them: I'm your mother, not your buddy. My job is to guide you as you go through this world until you are old enough to make it on your own. That means setting limits and reminding you when you don't adhere to them. Sass me once, good for you. Sass me twice, you're grounded. When I was a teenager and opened a fresh mouth, my parents took the phone out of the wall (can you imagine, a phone with a cord?). With my own teen and tween, the iPhone gets hidden away or the Xbox goes in the closet. And I mean business. There is no negotiating; you get it back when I say you get it back.

The key to making any and all of the above work is teamwork; your hubby has to be your VP, nodding his head, even when you say ridiculous things: "That's right, whatever Mommy says goes." You and your spouse may not agree 100 percent on every aspect of parenting, but you should *seem* like you do, at least to your kids. Mine try and pit us against each other: "But Mom, Dad said . . ." No, Dad didn't say it (if he did, he better take it back if he knows what's good for him). You have to parent in sync, backing each other up at all times. I tell my hubby that we are a team—it's us against them—and teammates stick together. Where would pitcher Noah Syndergaard be without closer Jeurys Familia? The Mets metaphor does wonders.

The bitch way to get kids to behave

A bitch does not let her children walk all over her. Kids can be demanding. Kids can be demonic. You can be a loving, devoted parent but still set ground rules and enforce them. If you're sick of having a daily showdown, there's a lot you can do to get your children in line.

Keep your cool. The more you yell, the less leverage you have. Stay in control despite your frustration, or it will turn into a shouting match worse than the presidential debates. If you can show your child that this is how you deal with disagreements, he'll pick up on your vibe and calm the hell down. Or he'll get so annoyed with your zombie-like presence, he'll vow to leave home as soon as he's eighteen. Either one works for me.

Hit pause. I find that most tantrums or fights happen when a kid is tired or hungry. Fix it fast. Offer a snack, a glass of milk, a nap—anything to encourage a cease-fire. After they (and you) have had a chance to refuel, you'll have a better chance of getting through to them once they're no longer hangry.

Start with a warning. Give your kids the opportunity to correct their own bad behavior before punishment is inflicted: "Blake,

I'll take away your dinner plate if you throw mashed potatoes at your brother again." Usually, I'll give my kids three chances— by the third strike, they're out. Now they know that you mean business and it's not just an idle threat. You go to bed without dinner . . . and you have to pay for the rug to be cleaned.

Kids need consequences. You can't just threaten to take away their phone; you have to follow through on it. If that results in tears or protests ("You're the meanest mom in the world and I hate you!"), then so be it. They'll remember what happens when they cross you, and they won't do it again. Just make sure the punishment fits the crime. If your son breaks his little sister's toy, I'm not sure a year of no TV is a valid consequence. Maybe have him play with her for an hour while you put your feet up and take a nap? I'm for any punishment that gives me a break! Likewise, you should reward good behavior: a gold star sticker on a chart is fine for some; mine prefer an iTunes gift card. Whatever works for you and your kids.

Be clear. Kids need to have their rules reinforced and modeled. If you're trying to teach them not to call each other names, don't refer to your hubby as "you lazy slob" in their presence (even if he is acting like one). Make sure everyone understands what is expected and tolerated in your home, then repeat it over and over again. I've discovered that most tweens and teens exhibit selective amnesia. Stick a Post-it on their heads if you have to: "Flush the toilet after you make a deposit."

Guilt them into it. Every child of a Jewish (or Catholic) mom knows the pain of guilt—it's torture as well as a great teaching tool. When your kid does something wrong, look them in the eye and say, "I'm very disappointed in you." When I do, my kids crumble. The last thing they want to do is make Mommy think they're less than spectacular. They want your applause! Allow them to wallow in it for a few minutes (even beg for your forgiveness) before you let them off the hook. I just channel my inner Nanadoll.

Manipulate the hell out of them. Don't they use their charms and dimples to twist us around their fingers? I've resorted to hiding healthy food in my daughter's meals ("It's not broccoli! It's a tree!"); bribing my son $10 to pack his own lunch and take his baseball bag to school; and hijacking my tween's technology ("The WiFi isn't working? Ya don't say!"). I am the queen of reverse psychology ("No, Jax, you don't have to study for your math test. You can just flunk it!) and scary stories ("When mommy was a little girl, I had a friend who *never* brushed her teeth, and they all fell out!"). A little mean? Maybe. Effective? One hundred percent!

A bitch-eye view of the world

I tell my kids all the time: be smart, be proactive, be prepared. Always expect the unexpected: your teacher will announce a pop quiz in Spanish class, and you won't see it coming. It's my job to teach you as best I can what I have learned in my forty-something years on this planet. Hopefully, you'll take notes and not *completely* ignore me.

My friend, celebrity stylist June Ambrose, puts it well: "Kids don't come with manuals, but they count on us to be their professors. I refer back to how I was raised textbook all the time. My mother was tough, but she was empathetic, and that taught me to care about others. She taught me that it was okay to be different and unapologetic for it. She was determined not to screw me up and 'over produce' me, but [instead] direct in a way that allowed my character to unfold and wow anyone who I came in contact with."

So, that's really my goal: to teach my kids that life is funny and slightly f'd up. The things that matter to you now will likely mean *nothing* down the road. The little shit who's bullying you in the school yard? He will disappear, and you won't even remember him when he comes up to you at your twentieth high school reunion. But it doesn't feel like that when you're a kid. It feels like every day is riddled with angst and endless issues and irritations. This is when you tell your kid what you know. You tell him/her:

Math doesn't matter. Unless you're planning on becoming an engineer, an accountant, or a nuclear physicist, in which case it matters a lot and you can worry less about English lit. But if your lifelong dream is to become a writer for Saturday Night Live, *a fashion designer, or a sports announcer for the Mets, it's okay to screw up an occasional prealgebra test. It isn't life-threatening. It's one quiz, one moment in a life that's going to be filled with lots of bigger moments. Don't let it rattle your confidence. Do what you can to fix the situation, then move on and do better next time.*

I can hear all those tiger moms out there hissing and booing me: "Grades count! School matters!" Of course, they do, but it doesn't matter *so much* that your kid needs to develop an anxiety disorder. Maybe you don't agree with me; maybe you are bent on having your kid go to Harvard. Your kid, your rules, so I'm not going to argue. But this is simply what I feel: I want my kids to be happy and healthy, period. So, in my opinion, a straight-A report card is nice, but not mandatory. I would rather them not be nervous wrecks all the time. I took earth science and calculus and stressed my way through both. Ask me if I use them today. Ask me if I wish I had known that little nugget of wisdom when I was in high school.

I know you're upset. I know this crisis feels ginormous right now, but I promise you, one day you won't care or remember the awful details. There are things in life worth crying about—trust me, I've experienced quite a few—but this isn't one of them. Be strong because I know you have it in you. As Nanadoll is fond of saying, "What doesn't kill ya makes ya stronger." She's not wrong (as much as I hate to admit that).

I am determined to raise kids that take a licking and keep on ticking. I wish growing up I knew what I know now. I wish I could have saved my tears for situations that really merited them. I wish I knew that every boyfriend who dumped me would become merely a humorous anecdote shared during a Girls'

Night Out. The hurdles that felt insurmountable were nothing more than stepping stones. So, this is what I want to arm my kids with: life can suck at times, but you can and will get through it if you grit your teeth and summon your inner superhero. Me? I'm Wonder Woman.

You've got a pretty good life—not everyone is so lucky. So stop complaining that things are unfair. I want you to think about how many people don't have what you have: a good school, a nice home, a loving family, vacations to Disneyworld, the latest iPhone. Seriously, things could be a lot worse, and you need to thank your lucky stars you've got a mom like me.

Grateful is not an option; it's something I insist that my kids feel. I want them to give a shit. I want them to give more than a shit. I may be a bitch, but I am a bighearted and generous one. I don't let a day go by without telling my nearest and dearest, "I love you." I don't tune out the evening world news because it doesn't happen in my backyard. I want to raise kids who are aware and care, so we talk about things that are going on around us, even if they're a little scary. We don't look away from the homeless guy begging for change on the subway; in fact, we give him some money and a few kind words. Empathy is a tool I want my kids to have. It helps you keep things in perspective and reminds you of what is really important in life.

Yes, I'm annoying. Pretty much everything—school, friends, parents—is a pain in the ass that you have to get through till you reach adulthood. Then you have to deal with bosses, husbands, and in-laws . . . but I digress. We all got through it, and you will, too. You can be annoyed all you want, but you can't fast-forward past being a kid.

Suck it up, buttercup. I'm sorry to say that not every moment of growing up is a party. Sometimes, you have to plow through what pisses you off to get to where you're going. How many boring classes did I have to sit through to graduate? How many mind-numbing jobs did I take till I landed on my dream one?

How many frogs did I kiss till I picked out my prince? I want my kids to understand that growing up isn't easy peasy, lemon squeezy. I tell them, "Things *will* bug the crap out of you. You're entitled to feel that way. But just know it's not getting any better for at least a few years until you can do what you want without my permission." That's when they'll truly appreciate me and wish I was still nagging them to put on clean underwear. Because you know they'll forget.

Set them free

I also remind myself that it is my job to create a human being capable of existing untethered from the umbilical cord. My friend, Dr. Robi Ludwig, author of *Your Best Age Is Now* says: "Eventually, children will grow up to live their own independent lives. And this is the way it should be. Moms need to love their child, but also realize their job is to raise them to fly and to be independent beings."

A bitch knows when to back off; part of her power is instilling power in others. So, yes, Blakey, you can pour your own apple juice in the morning. Okay, Ollie, you don't need me hovering when you hang upside down on the monkey bars. And fine, Jax, feel free to make plans with your pals without me calling their moms and arranging. Good for you all for taking ownership of your lives and forging your identities. I try to give my kids lots of choices. Where do you want to go? What do you want to eat? But there is never an endless pool of possibilities, because that is just asking for trouble and arguments. It's more either/or. Pizza or pasta? The park or the zoo? And you have to convince your fellow siblings to get on board. This allows them to feel in control of the situation (when really I am), and when things don't go as well as they had hoped ("The polar bears are sleeping!" "My pizza is burnt!"), they've made their choices and have to live with them. This greatly reduces the number of temper tantrums. They may be disappointed, but they're not gonna admit they were wrong and should have gone with what was behind curtain number two.

If they try to do something new but don't succeed, you should always praise them for the effort. Bite your tongue if it's a train wreck; you want them to take risks, don't you? And if they're learning a new skill—in Blakey's case brushing her teeth—try not to swoop in and make corrections. Never do for a kid what they can do for themselves, which is almost anything. Just know to leave extra time for your toddler to work though his/her new task. Mine will spend thirty minutes playing in the sink with her pretty pink toothbrush, and I have to resist the urge to grab it out of her hand and just be done with it.

And finally, forget the idea of *perfect*. No kid is perfect; no mom is perfect (although bitches come *very* close). Truly, I despise the word *perfect*. We all screw up and that's okay. Never compare yourself to any other family—as easy as that is to do with everyone posting adorable pics on Facebook. Be you; encourage your kids to be themselves. Embrace the crazy, because without it, we'd all be Stepford mamas. Laugh at your flaws and your kids' kookiness. Weird, in this bitch's opinion, is wonderful.

How to throw a bitchin' b-day party for your child

I have a lot of thoughts on this topic, probably because I started out in PR and planned loads of events, and I love to be creative. I believe you don't ignore a single detail of a party; it's the little things that add up and make it special. For Blakey's second birthday, we had Minnie Mouse make an appearance and did a matching Minnie cake, paper goods, and favors. Ollie, my budding Broadway star, had a theater-themed b-day, complete with a Playbill-covered cake. So, yes, I like to go above and beyond; that's just me.

Here are some words of caution: at the end of the day, it's not *your* day, it's your child's day. Do not throw a party trying to impress people (i.e., the snooty mom bunch). And resist coming down with what my friend Lindsey Peers, owner of The Craft Studio in New York City, has dubbed PDC, Party Day Crazy.

Lindsey admits, "I have been guilty of PDC before, and it is easy to do. It is when a normally very chill and relaxed mom snaps over the stress of the party day arriving. Enjoy, who cares if your shipment of Shopkins T-shirts is arriving [the day after the party], you can hand deliver [them] and extend the celebration! A cool and collected mom, not a frazzled and stressed one, will leave the happiest of impressions on the b-day boy or girl, and that is what this is all about."

Make the celebration personal and special for your kid; that should be your guiding force. Because no one is going to remember the six-tier *Star Wars* cake. But your child will remember the love in the room. My friend Marni Konner, creator and owner of Little Maestros, says it best: "Don't blink! The party will be over before you know it. Stay in the moment and savor as much as possible."

The dos and don'ts of throwing a bitchin' b-day bash

I asked Dylan Lauren, owner of Dylan's Candy Bar and mom to twins, to share her secrets for doing it right. She's the most creative mom mogul I know—and also one of the most organized.

Do plan early! Locking in a date that's most convenient for you and contacting important guests before the invitations arrive helps avoid unwanted stress.

Don't try to accommodate everyone's schedule. It's hard enough to get your family's ducks in a row, so just do the best you can.

Do set a realistic budget. It will help when planning all details, from the location to the food, with wiggle room for unexpected extras.

Don't overextend your finances. Do your research to avoid feeling pressured to make rush decisions, spending more than necessary. There's no reason to compare yourself to someone else; it's the personal touches that matter.

Do prescreen and book your entertainment immediately. Have some back-up dates available if they're the focal point of the event, and use their direct line over an agent's if you can.

Don't skip the in-person research. You don't need to book an entertainer, but be sure to see him/her in person if you are to see how they jive.

Do shop party locations like a pro. Make a short list of must-haves and nice-to-haves to help you narrow it down.

Don't get too critical. Visit your top two to three spots to ensure your research aligns, and then trust your gut and eyes! Look into untapped locations—kids prefer variety over the same old places.

Do discuss your needs with the on-site coordinator. Find out if there are any discounted off-peak hours or days to help keep costs down.

Don't feel inelegant asking about options. It's perfectly fine to inquire about discounts; venues often use them to retain new customers.

Do involve your kids in the planning process. Allow them to pick a theme or let them choose between cupcakes and cake. (It's a great learning lesson, too!)

Don't let your child dictate every detail. You handle the big stuff and encourage your kids to have fun with the smaller decisions.

Do explore DIY decor and games. It's a great bonding activity for the whole family, and it's fun to inspire guests with homemade talents.

Don't obsess over every detail. Your party doesn't need to be photo-shoot worthy; it just needs to be fun! Don't go crazy trying to recreate your Pinterest board.

Do recruit family and friends to help. Do you have a friend who's crafty or loves to bake? It's a great excuse to spend time together.

Don't wait until the last minute, when you're swamped. People have their own priorities, but you'd be surprised how willing they are to help if you give them a heads-up.

Do make a note on invitations inquiring about allergies. This will help to ensure you have some options for your guests to freely enjoy without worrying. Be sure the food or candy handlers are educated on allergy concerns and on avoiding contamination.

Don't discount dietary constraints. Though it seems a new allergy concern is popping up every day, it's better to err on the side of caution.

Do personalize it! Set up a small candy and dessert bar stocked with treats that are your child's favorites. Try creating a custom ribbon or sticker with a fun image of your child or party logo on it.

Don't feel like the party itself is the gift. It's always a nice touch to show guests how much you appreciate their attendance and remind them of the special day you shared.

Bitch of the Day

"My son loves to make trouble. Today, he flushed his little brother's favorite Lego figure down the toilet."

Put your foot down before you have a flood: "No more wreaking havoc on our home!" What's behind the bad behavior? Is he bored? Jealous of your little one? Making mischief to get your attention? Sit him down and try to get to the heart of where his actions are coming from. Then find a fitting punishment for the crime. I say he has to build the entire Death Star out of Legos for his little bro, even if it takes him a week and a gazillion Legos to do it. Make him apologize to his sibling, crack open his piggy bank to buy him a new one, and swear he'll never do it again.

STEP 9
WHIP YOUR HUBBY

"When you have a baby, love is automatic, when you get married, love is earned."

—Marie Osmond

My husband, Brian, and I have been married for sixteen years of bliss! We never, ever fight, the sex is hotter than ever, and every day is just perfect and magical!

Okay, now you *know* I'm pulling your leg. Our marriage is like most: a roller coaster of highs and lows with lots of midlevel periods in between. But when the universe has thrown us curve balls (three kids, changing jobs, the deaths of both our dads in the past four years), we've managed to cling to each other and weather the storms—the sign of a strong union. They ain't kidding when they say, "for better or worse, for richer or poorer, in sickness and in health . . ." If you've been married as long as we've been, all of those conditions come into play. Marriage is work, *hard* work, and only the toughest survive. So, Bri, it's a good thing you've got a bitch in your corner!

We met way back when through a mutual friend. I thought he was handsome, tall (a prerequisite, since I'm five-foot nine), nice, funny, and kind. What more did I want at twenty-five? Our fairy tale wedding proposal was even written up in *Brides* magazine: Brian told me that we were going to Cort Theatre, where we had met two years earlier, to see a preview of a new Broadway play. He picked me up that night outside of my office, and he was late as usual. By the time we rushed into the lobby just after eight o'clock, an usher informed us that the performance had already started, so he would not let us in to see the show. I was tired and soaking wet from the rain, and I just wanted to go home and dry out. Brian got angry and told the usher that we had to see the show for work purposes. After a few minutes of bickering, the usher agreed to take us to our seats. When the doors opened, I was shocked: the theater was empty except for what looked like hundreds of flowers. Brian then handed me a Playbill with a picture of us inside that read, "Elyssa and Brian Get Engaged." He got down on one knee and asked me to marry him.

After such a fine performance, my answer was most definitely yes! We had a big, beautiful wedding followed by a honeymoon in Hawaii. A few years later, our first son, Jackson, was born, and the rest is history. We don't always see eye-to-eye, and we don't always agree on how to raise our kids. For every wonderful moment (the birth of your children, your son's bar mitzvah, a fabulous family vacation), there are also the bad ones. There's the time your kid throws up all night (on you) or your father becomes ill with cancer. Marriage is the sum of all those parts. You can't prepare for the scary, sad times; you can only promise each other to do your very best.

I have many friends who are divorced, and I don't judge—it's your right to be happy, and if you're happier apart, so be it. But I do think, as a couple, you ask the question: are we in this for the long haul? If the answer is yes, then you fight. You fight really hard to keep the fires burning, the communication flowing, and the fun alive and kickin'. You don't give up—not on your life together and not on each other as individuals. You take the good with the bad and remind yourself why you fell in love ten, fifteen, or twenty years ago. It's still there, you just gotta look for it.

A long time ago, I decided that my marriage would be a partnership of equals. I want my kids to see through their dad's example the way a wife deserves to be treated. They will model it one day. Blakey will choose a great guy to walk down the aisle with, and he better kiss her ass. I know a lot of women who slip into a passive mode. They let the husband be the breadwinner and decision maker. One guy even informed his wife, "He who makes the gold makes the rules." Sorry, Fred Flintstone, the caveman era is over. He who makes the gold should put it on his wife's wrist, neck, and earlobes. We deserve it. We *more* than deserve it.

To be fair—and to give the guy a chance to say something—I asked Brian to help me out on this chapter. "Tell me what it is all men want from their wives," I asked him. On a plane to Vegas, en route to a biz trip (see "Does Absence Make the Heart Grow Fonder?" on page 103), he wrote and emailed me a pithy list. I have to say, I kind of agree—he hit the nail on the head. But what most men aren't prepared for is how a bitch will interpret those five basic needs. Careful what you wish for . . .

Hubby necessity #1: Sex

Well, duh. I have never met a guy not governed by his penis. How important is it? It truly depends on the man. Some need it desperately and ask for it constantly, usually when you're ready to drop from exhaustion. But if you *don't* deliver, they feel neglected, wounded, deprived, and you won't stop hearing about it. Others are not as amorous but require the occasional stroking of the ego (or other things) to make them feel like they're in step with their peers.

Experts tell me that men and women need sex for different reasons. Males produce testosterone, which makes sex a biological necessity. The sperm builds up, and it needs to be released—kind of like when we were nursing and our boobs swelled with milk. It felt damn good to get it outta there! For females, it's less about biology and more about emotions. It's a connection, a way of expressing love, devotion, and appreciation. A quickie once in a while is fine, but what most women want is the stuff that romance novels are made of. Men don't seem to get this concept. We want to be swept off our feet. We want to be told we're beautiful. We want to be caressed, not groped, petted like a dog, or kneaded like a ball of pizza dough.

I don't care how much other couples brag, or how many studies say that married people get it on more than singletons.

Most couples hit a dry spell now and then or have problems with performance. It's normal, but usually one (or both) of the partners isn't too happy about it. As a couple, you need to figure out why you're not making whoopee like you used to.

Ouch, it hurts! After pushing two or three kids out of your lady parts, things are stretched, bruised, and scarred. It can take weeks, maybe even months, for you to get back in the saddle and feel "normal" again, and some women suffer even longer than that. Even if you haven't recently given birth, things down below can be a bit sensitive, especially if they're not getting a regular workout. Dryness becomes a big issue when you hit your forties— it's like all of a sudden, thanks to fluctuations in estrogen, it's the Sahara Desert down there. Experts say to do your Kegel exercises daily, lubricate well, and take it slow and easy.

I'm too tired. Honey, I hear ya. Most nights, my head hits the pillow and I'm out like a light. According to WebMD, recent polls show that 50 percent of couples skip sex because they're too tired. In these cases, nighttime may no longer be the right time for you. You may need to try sex in the a.m., after a nap, or when the kids are at baseball practice. If it's important to you (and it should be), fit it into your schedule earlier in the day. Where there's a will, there's a way.

He's not a team player. Okay, this is a big passion killer for a lot of bitchy mamas: bottled-up resentment. You're mad/disgusted with his lack of cooperation; you feel like you're the one doing all the work when it comes to family and home. He doesn't pitch in as much as you'd like, and it's hard not to hate his guts for it. One friend told me her hubby strolls in at 6:00 p.m., kicks off his shoes, pours himself a drink, and relaxes on the couch while she slaves over a hot stove, helps her tween with his homework, and struggles to get their toddler twins bathed and ready for bed. In this bitch's book, that doesn't happen. You're tired? You had a hard day at work? You should see what *I* had to deal with today! Raising a family is a full-time job, and a lot of moms have an office job on top of it. So, if you want sex tonight, sweetheart, get a clue: set the table, entertain the kids, fold the laundry. I have one word for you: choreplay.

It's never about me. I hear this complaint a lot from my fellow moms: he wants it when he wants it, not when I do. What happened to fulfilling my needs and putting a smile on my face? When did sex become a dictatorship or a means of control? As a bitch, it's your duty to nip this situation in the bud: he doesn't get to call the shots in the bedroom. You decide together, and you make it about you as a couple, not him as king. You know what happens to most kings, right? They get overthrown or offed.

This also leads to a bigger issue: men who try to dominate in a marriage. It takes a very strong woman to live with and love a guy with a healthy ego and a hint of control freak. As a bitch, you must assert yourself and declare your independence! Tell yourself, and then him:

- I love who I am and I don't have to change for anyone.
- I am proud of my success, my brains, and my talent.
- I will state my opinion, whether you ask for it or not.
- I don't have to "check in" with you or get your permission to do things. I'm a grown-up.
- I have a right to my own space with no interruptions.
- I can spend money responsibly as I see fit.
- I have an equal say in all family matters.

Hubby necessity #2: Great communication

Sometimes I feel like I'm talking to a brick wall; no one in my home hears me, or I have to repeat the same thing over and over and send an email confirmation. Most men don't make the best listeners, but they are really adept at tuning out noise, namely, your nagging them. There is a better way to get your point across.

- Everything is on the table, meaning no subject is taboo, including sex (or your lack of it), how much his mom is driving you nuts, or the fact that he needs to pop a Mentos at this moment. No changing the subject; no avoiding the issue. Honesty above all.

- Say it with love. If you have to share any of the above, make sure it comes from a place of kindness. Prefacing any gripe with Sweetheart, Honey Bear, or Lambchop helps (unless you gag when saying it). But seriously, be gentle, not vicious.
- Look on the bright side. Be positive, even if you're pointing out problems. What can you do together to make this better? What's a good way to tackle it and put it behind you?
- Talk less, listen more. Once you've aired your grievance, give him a chance to respond in turn. Hear him out; maybe he has a damn good explanation.
- Time it right. When he's had a bad day at work or your kids are a captive audience is probably not the best time to have a discussion. Wait till you two are alone, relaxed, and you have his undivided attention—not when he's trying to watch a Mets game.
- Talk, don't yell. Disagreements don't have to turn into shouting matches. Stay calm and collected and ask him to do the same. There's no issue that can be solved easier at a louder volume.
- Move on. Like the chick from *Frozen* sings, "Let it go." Once you've said your peace and he's responded, don't beat the issue to death. Maybe it will take several other sit-downs to fix things; that's okay. For the moment, leave it be.

Hubby necessity #3: Occasional peace and quiet

I get it: men need their space. Some actually require a man cave to chill in. Mine just needs an hour to nap without me nagging and the kids jumping on his head. Can't say I blame him for trying to tune out. If I could, I would! It's also not a bad thing if occasionally your husband wants to go out with the boys or veg in a hammock in the backyard. There's nothing in the marriage vows that says you have to be together 24/7. I'm of the mind-set that in order to stay together, a couple needs to spend time apart.

Does Absence Make the Heart Grow Fonder?

My husband has to travel a lot for business. In the beginning, I wasn't too happy about this fact. Besides missing him, it made me really anxious. What would I do if I blew a fuse in our apartment? What if one of the kids came down with a stomach bug? What if I came down with a stomach bug? What if something caught fire? I never signed up to be a single mom of three! But then, gradually, I got used to it and realized how I could handle any crisis without him to swoop in and rescue me. Being apart from him actually built me up. It didn't damage our marriage; in fact, I actually appreciated my hubby more when he got home.

A 2013 study in the *Journal of Communication* found that couples in long-distance relationships actually have more meaningful interactions than those who see each other daily. I believe it; Brian looks really good to me when I haven't seen him in a week. I forget all the stuff he does to normally bug the crap out of me and welcome him back with open arms. My mom friends tell me the same: after being alone with their kids for several days, they're jumping for joy when their husbands return. Same goes for my working mom pals who also travel for business. After logging in miles apart, being back with the hubby feels great. And there's something really hot about welcome home sex—it's like rediscovering each other all over again.

Yes, schedule in plenty of quality time for two, but also allow for separateness. You don't have to like doing all the same things; it's healthy to go off on your own and then come back refreshed. Some of my friends strongly disagree with me. They think that giving your hubby a break invites him to check out altogether (out of sight, out of mind), or worse, cheat on you. I think you know your husband best and how much "leash" you can give him. Maybe a Vegas weekend is too much, but a golf afternoon with his frat brothers is just right. Just remember, what goes for him goes for you as well. If he wants to sleep in till 11:00 a.m. this weekend, the next one is yours.

Hubby necessity #4: A best friend

Being married to someone isn't just about love, sex, and paying pediatrician bills. It's about friendship, a deep and meaningful bond. It's having each other's back, and supporting your spouse whenever he/she feels most fragile and vulnerable. Think about the things you love about your best gal pals: they make you feel good about yourself; they talk you off a ledge; they know your flaws and love you anyway; they tell you the truth when no one else will. Same goes for your hubby. This is what he wants and expects from you. He also wants someone to have fun with, who laughs at his jokes even if they're not funny. He wants you to be proud of him, even brag a little. Friends do that for friends.

He wants you to be loyal and to give him the same get-out-of-jail-free card you would give a BFF. If he has a bad day and takes it out on you, he needs you to forgive and forget. Just remind him that to have a good friend, you have to be one, too.

Hubby necessity #5: Mutual respect

Hell, yeah! This one might actually be at the top of my list for what wives want. I've talked a lot about how resentment breeds a bad marriage. Well, it starts with a lack of respect. You may not always agree with your spouse, but you have to respect his/her opinions, plain and simple. No bad-mouthing, no berating, no belittling. When you respect your partner, you understand that he/she is not your mirror image. You are both individual human beings, not playthings, punching bags, or afterthoughts. Respect is treating someone the way you want to be treated. It's not dissing them in front of the kids (or in public). It's showing kindness and regard for their crazy relatives (because we all have them), their upbringing, and their traditions. It's honoring who they are and what they do and not making them feel like chopped liver (as Nanadoll would say). Care what they think and feel; ask, don't assume. If you lose respect, love usually follows, so make it a priority.

Little white lies. What *shouldn't* you tell him?

I know I preach that honesty is always the best policy, and I mean it. That said, there are a few scenarios when it's simply TMI. Don't tell him . . .

- how much your kid's after-school activities *really* cost. It will only make his blood pressure go up. If he asks, it's okay to round down.
- that you have diarrhea, gas, or excruciating period cramps. What happens in the bathroom stays in the bathroom!
- that your mother thinks he's a moron. Yeah, that won't go over well on the holidays.
- that you've put on five pounds. If he didn't notice, no need to broadcast it.
- that he's put on five pounds . . . even if you notice.
- that your high school boyfriend asked to follow you on Facebook. Water under the bridge.
- that one of your girlfriends is cheating on her husband with a silver-haired fox. You'll make him wonder if you're envious (okay, maybe just a little).

Bitch of the Day

"My husband snores all night like a buzz saw and I can't get any sleep!"

I assume you've tried everything: Breathe Right strips, snore pillows, mouth guards, nose plugs, ear plugs, kicking him in the shins. If you don't want to sleep in separate rooms (I don't recommend it for the sake of your sex life), then suggest he see a sleep doc. You need to get to the bottom of what's causing all that ruckus. Did he gain weight? Does he suffer from sleep apnea? If he's resistant to seeing a specialist, remind him that sleep apnea is actually dangerous and can lead to high blood pressure, heart disease, diabetes, and a host of other health problems. That should scare him into it.

STEP 10
JUST SAY NO

*I know not everyone will like me, but this is who I am,
so if you don't like it, tough!*

—*Britney Spears*

Setting your limits and boundaries is essential if you're going to be a bitch. You won't get a gold star for being a pleaser; you'll just get a migraine. I find the more I do for others, the more people see it as an opening to take advantage of me. Give an inch, they take a yard. So, while I'm all for generosity and community service, I'm not for every dirty job no one else is willing to take on. I used to be. I was the sap everyone knew to call for a last-minute favor: "Oh, Lyss, she's a peach! She'll do it." And I did—till I had no time left in my day for anything I needed to do. I was everybody's free labor and patsy. Then I wised up: where was this getting me? People didn't like me more for it—they saw me as a sucker. So I stopped, cold turkey. One day, I looked someone in the eye and said, "No." Actually, I think I said, "No f'in' way." But the message was the same: thanks, but no thanks, find someone else.

Just because I work from home doesn't mean I need to work for *you* from home. Do I have "pushover" stamped on my forehead? Didn't think so. I'm very selective about the use of my time and energy. I know a lot of moms have trouble asserting themselves when people ask for favors. Not me, not now. I look 'em straight in the eye, smile, and apologize for having to pass. There's nothing you can say or do to change my mind.

Saying no is incredibly liberating—like throwing off the shackles of indentured servitude. I say no constantly, just for the fun of it. "Mom, can I have another cookie?" No. "Honey, did you see my shoes?" No. "Lyss, can you meet me tomorrow so I can get your opinion on my new bathroom tiles?" No. If I had more time/energy/interest, I might not answer in the negative. But I don't, so I won't. My time is precious, so I'm not going to waste a second. I'm also not going to give in just because someone is whining. (Brian, that goes for you, too.) I have absolutely no trouble being a no-slinging bitch in any situation that merits it.

Saying no to your kids

If you're already putting step seven into practice, then you're getting quite a bit of practice. Say it too much to a child and it loses its impact; they assume the answer will always be the same, so they stop asking and just *do*. Kids need rules and limits. They need to learn how to deal with disappointment, frustration, and delayed gratification. Isn't that what adult life is all about? I've learned that a flat-out no is less effective. I do the no/yes thing: "No, you can't punch your brother, but, yes, you can change the channel to your show. Let's take turns." Or "No, you can't have a cupcake now, but, yes, you can have one after you finish your veggies." Also, mind your tone: if you bark, it's like waving a red flag in your kid's face. This makes mommy mad, so let's do it again! Instead, keep your cool and stand by your refusal. If you waver, they'll smell fear! No is no—no backpedaling.

Saying no to a friend

Friends ask us to do the damnedest things, and because we don't want to hurt anyone's feelings, we often cave. But you don't have to; dole out your favors carefully. A woman I know wound up throwing a wedding for her BFF's daughter in her backyard—eight-piece orchestra and all—when her pal whined she had no room. Another agreed to go on Match.com to stalk her friend's ex-husband, only to discover he was gay. Imagine having to break *that* news.

Friends know we have a hard time saying no to them; they count on it. I have some strict policies: I don't lend friends money—that's a recipe for disaster. Ask me to spot you a ten and I'm fine with it, but I'm not writing you a check for your child's summer camp. I also don't fake employment applications for them (I have never been nor will I ever will be your boss) or help them fudge a tax return (and, believe me, I've been asked!). Don't ever compromise your morals or your bank account, no matter how great the chum. If they're a good friend, they'll understand that you're uncomfortable and won't hold it against you. If they do, they've just shown their true colors. Unfriend them on LinkedIn.

Saying no to your school

I dread the first day of the school year—it's when the current PTA officers descend on us like vultures in the halls or the yard, roping us into volunteering for the carnival, the bake sale, the safety committee. A new year means new blood. I keep my head down and avoid eye contact. They can't get you if you don't engage. Beyond that, I learned the power of the polite turndown with a little excuse on the side. "Oh, I would love to man the face-painting booth this year, but I'm already committed to taking my mother-in-law to a matinee and lunch. Maybe next time!" I find the more specific you are, the less they can poke holes in your excuse. If I say, "I'm busy," I open it up to an avalanche of questions: "Busy doing what? Is it *that* important? Isn't your child's school more important? Don't you want to be a good mother?" No one messes with the mother-in-law defense; they feel your pain. And speaking of in-laws . . .

Saying no to your hubby's mom

A delicate situation, to say the least. Piss her off and she will hold it against you for the rest of your married life. She will tell your husband, "I told you so." So, I never make my nos about me—they're always about his or her grandkids. "We'd love for you to come visit this weekend, but your son promised his boys he was taking them to a game at Citi Field. Isn't that the sweetest?" I've learned to pick and choose my battles wisely with my MIL. Basically, it's not worth it to challenge her; your husband will always take his mom's side, because she gave birth to him. It may have been fifty years ago, but he hasn't forgotten. Turn a deaf ear to the endless critiques: of course she raised her children better and her brisket is never tough. But I'll tell you what is tough: a bitch. Smile, act grateful for any advice, and show the ultimate respect and reverence. But in the end, do whatever you want. (Don't tell my mother-in-law I said that!)

Saying no to *your* mother

Even worse than the above. Oh, the guilt! My mom is a master of manipulation. Seriously, the woman could run for president of the United States and win. As she's gotten on in years (she won't admit how many), she's also become more demanding. My phone rings several times a day with questions, concerns, and the need for breaking news. "What is Blakey wearing? Does her bow match her shoes? What are you making for dinner tonight?" All very important info, I assure you. And the woman can't email and wait for the answer—it has to be over the phone with an instantaneous response. She's a widow, so I do cut her some slack. I know she misses my dad and needs to feel needed. I need her, too. I need her empathy, advice, and unconditional love. My mom is my biggest cheerleader; I just wish she didn't cheer so loudly all the time!

Bitch of the Day

"My sister asked me to be the matron of honor at her third wedding. I've done this twice before—isn't someone else available?"

I say you've done your sisterly duty (and then some). If there are no other siblings to stand at the altar with her, then suggest she ask a friend, coworker, even take an ad out on Craigslist, for God's sake. The role of matron is fraught with anxiety, financial obligations, and endless busywork, as you well know, because this ain't your first rodeo. Are you supposed to throw her a shower (again!)? Are you supposed to buy a hideous gown (again!)? Say no, but add "thank you" after it. Tell her you've got a ton of work and family commitments and don't feel right not being able to give her wedding 110 percent. Don't let her suck you in. If you say yes this time, what happens when she's on wedding number four, five, or six? Think of it as a bad habit, like smoking. You have to stop at some point for the sake of your health.

CONCLUSION
Congrats! You're a Bitchy Mama!

"We need to understand that there is no formula for how women should lead their lives. That is why we must respect the choices that each woman makes for herself and her family. Every woman deserves the chance to realize her God-given potential."

—Hillary Clinton

You've studied and completed all ten steps in the program. Now you need to go forth and be fierce! You must maintain your bitchiness at all times and on all occasions, even when a new kid comes along and you're back to square one. Make yourself a checklist and glance at it from time to time to make sure you're on track. As a bitch, you must always:

- Believe in your strength, your smarts, and your talent.
- Assert yourself at all times; no one puts baby in the corner.
- Set boundaries and make sure no one steps over the line.
- Reclaim your mojo—be a hot mama and look the part from head to toe.
- Put yourself first: eat healthy, exercise, take time-outs.
- Be clear with your family about what you want/need from them and accept nothing less.
- Surround yourself with people who think like you and aren't afraid to grow a pair.
- Say no if a task or a favor is too much to ask of you.
- Make some noise if you're not being heard—like Katy Perry sings, "Roar!"
- Be a leader, not a follower. A player, not a spectator.
- Inspire and light a fire under those who could use a little boost of bitch in their lives. Spread it around!

And now, let's review and see how much you remember!

Quiz: What would a bitch do?

1. Your husband comes home from work and puts his feet up on the couch to relax. You:
    a) offer to rub his tired, aching tootsies
    b) put your feet up, too—guess dinner will make itself

2. Your babysitter insists you order her a gourmet lunch. You:
    a) hand her a menu and your credit card
    b) enlighten her that if Lean Cuisine frozen ravioli is good enough for you, it's good enough for her

3. Your son's teacher calls to tell you he's been misbehaving. You:
    a) apologize profusely and offer to ground him for life
    b) suggest that perhaps her class control isn't up to snuff, but you'd be more than happy to come in and show her how it's done

4. Your boss hits you up with a ridiculously impossible deadline. You:
    a) stay up all night for the next week: who needs sleep?
    b) Say, "Hmmm, I wonder how the ACLU would feel about this? Maybe I should just give them a call."

5. Your mother calls to tell you she's feeling a little achy … again. You:
    a) offer to take her to the ER (again). You can't be too careful!
    b) suggest she find another hobby besides hypochondria. How about mahjong?

Answer key:

Mostly As—Your inner bitch still needs a bit of work. Go back and read some of the steps again for a quick refresher. #imnobodysdoormat

All Bs—Brava! You've graduated with flying colors, and I'm proud to consider you a member of my bitch brigade. Keep up the good work, woman!

Why We All Need to Be Bitches

In case your friends and family don't get it (or you occasionally forget), here's a reminder of why being a bitch is not just a good thing, but a *great* thing.

Bitches are honest—with themselves and with others. You can always count on them for a truthful answer, an untainted opinion, advice that you may not want to hear but *need* to hear.

Bitches speak their minds. They don't back down from a bully (I'm still with Hil . . .). They call it like they see it, and they never censor themselves for fear of being unpopular.

Bitches have killer confidence. They strut around like they own the place—and they usually do. They never question or doubt themselves because they *know* themselves and their fabulosity.

Bitches don't care what you think. They don't want or seek your approval. They do what they want when they want without asking permission.

Bitches never say "I'm sorry." They don't apologize for being who they are or what they do. If you don't like it, I'm sorry . . . for you!

Bitches love themselves. They are comfortable in their own skin and don't give a rat's ass if they have cellulite.

Bitches embrace their femininity. They don't have to act like a man (or look like one) to exert their power. They do it in four-inch heels.

Bitches are happy . . . and healthy . . . and a helluva lotta fun to be around. They exude positivity, energy, and light and inspire everyone around them to be better, brighter, and bolder.

Bitches are smart. They don't rest on their laurels or allow themselves to get complacent or even bored. They strive to keep growing, learning, and evolving.

Bitches know no boundaries. There is nothing you can do to deter them from their path or goal.

Bitches run the show. And they should be running the world (at the very least, this country). They exude strength, courage, and determination in everything they do.

_____

_____

_____

_____

_____

_____

_____

_____

_____

_____

_____

_____

_____

_____

_____

_____

_____

_____

"There's nothing a man can do, that I can't do better and in heels."

—Ginger Rogers

Motherhood Is a B#tch

_____

_____

_____

_____

_____

_____

_____

_____

_____

_____

_____

_____

_____

_____

_____

_____

_____

_____

_____

_____

_____

_____

"The thing women have yet to learn is nobody gives you power. You just take it."
—Roseanne Barr

Motherhood Is a B#tch

_____

_____

_____

_____

_____

_____

_____

_____

_____

_____

_____

_____

_____

_____

_____

_____

_____

_____

_____

_____

_____

_____

_____

"Being a bitch means . . . I stand up for myself and my beliefs. I stand up for those I love, I speak my mind, think my own thoughts or do things my way.
—Britney Spears

Motherhood Is a B#tch

_____

_____

_____

_____

_____

_____

_____

_____

_____

_____

_____

_____

_____

_____

_____

_____

_____

_____

_____

_____

_____

_____

"These days, I strive to be a bitch, because not being one sucks. Not being a bitch means not having your voice heard."

—Margaret Cho

Motherhood Is a B#tch

_____

_____

_____

_____

_____

_____

_____

_____

_____

_____

_____

_____

_____

_____

_____

_____

_____

_____

_____

_____

_____

_____

"Who runs the world? Girls."

—Beyoncé Knowles

Motherhood Is a B#tch

"There are some people who still feel threatened by strong women. That's their problem. It's not mine."

—Gloria Allred

Motherhood Is a B#tch

_____
_____
_____
_____
_____
_____
_____
_____
_____
_____
_____
_____
_____
_____
_____
_____
_____
_____
_____
_____
_____

"I'm tough, I'm ambitious, and I know exactly what I want. If that makes me a bitch, okay."

—Madonna

Motherhood Is a B#tch

_____

_____

_____

_____

_____

_____

_____

_____

_____

_____

_____

_____

_____

_____

_____

_____

_____

_____

_____

_____

"When a man gives his opinion, he's a man. When a woman gives her opinion, she's a bitch."

—Bette Davis

Motherhood Is a B#tch

_____

_____

_____

_____

_____

_____

_____

_____

_____

_____

_____

_____

_____

_____

_____

_____

_____

_____

_____

_____

_____

"To be a bitch or not to be a bitch, that is the question."

—Shannen Doherty

Motherhood Is a B#tch

_____

_____

_____

_____

_____

_____

_____

_____

_____

_____

_____

_____

_____

_____

_____

_____

"I found my inner Bitch and ran with her."

—Courtney Love

Motherhood Is a B#tch

_____

_____

_____

_____

_____

_____

_____

_____

_____

_____

_____

_____

_____

_____

_____

_____

_____

_____

_____

_____

_____

_____

"Here's to strong women. May we know them. May we be them. May we raise them."

—Unknown

ACKNOWLEDGMENTS

A very special thank you to all the *fabULyss* women and men who took time out of their busy days to submit to this book: Rebecca Minkoff, Kelly Rutherford, Jenny Hutt, Erika Katz, Sasha Charnin Morrison, Aliza Licht, June Ambrose, Dr. Robi Ludwig, Fred DeVito, Elisabeth Halfpapp, Laura Geller, Warren Tricomi, Tanya Zuckerbrot, Keri Glassman, Jené Luciani, Barbara Reich, Tiffany Keriakos, Karen Kreitzer, Veronica Webb, Alison Brod, and Dylan Lauren.

To Sheryl Berk, my *fabULyss* and fierce friend and confidant, thank you for the tireless laughter, tears, and hours of sharing real-life stories that no one else would believe. I could not have written this book without you, so thank you for making it a reality.

Thank you, Jill Kargman, for writing the foreword, for your honesty, and for showing all the other *real* mothers out there that they are not alone.

To my editor, Brooke Rockwell, thank you for your tireless hard work on making this book what it is today. You understood my vision from the start and allowed my voice to be heard.

A very special thank-you to my friends and the support of the divamoms community. Thank you for allowing me to keep it all real, the tears, the joy, the laughter, the MOMentum.

ABOUT THE AUTHORS

Lyss Stern: Stern is "the mommy acknowledgments whisperer," columnist, and a "mompreneur." She created Divalysscious Moms (divamoms.com) as a way to get her groove back after giving birth to her first child and help other mothers find themselves postbaby. Today, it is the premier network and event company for the New York area's well-heeled moms. Stern lives in New York City with her husband, their three children, and their dog.

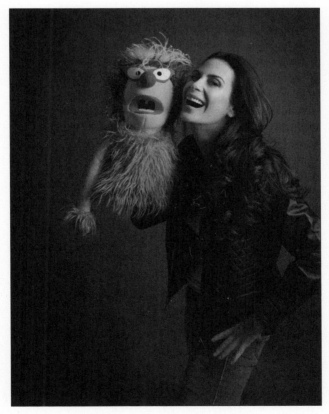

Photo by Lindsay May for Classic Kids Photography

Sheryl Berk: Berk is a *New York Times* best-selling author, founding editor in chief of *Life & Style Weekly*, and senior entertainment editor for *A&E Biography* and *McCall's.* She has collaborated with celebs on their memoirs/lifestyle books, and is coauthor (with her daughter) of a best-selling children's chapter book series. Berk lives in New York City with her husband and daughter.

Jill Kargman: Kargman is a born-and-bred New Yorker, age 41 (yes, she embraces her real age), who is not afraid to dish about life on the Upper East Side. She is a *New York Times* best-selling author and creator and star of Bravo TV's *Odd Mom Out.* Her newest book is titled *Sprinkle Glitter on My Grave.*

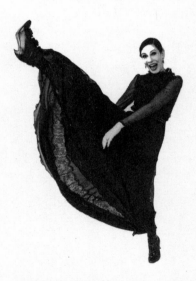

Photo by Deborah Feingold